Quick Reference to the
MANUAL OF CLINICAL PSYCHOPHARMACOLOGY

Contents

Manual of Clinical Psychopharmacology

Alan F. Schatzberg, M.D.
Jonathan O. Cole, M.D.

McLean Hospital
Belmont, Massachusetts

Harvard Medical School
Boston, Massachusetts

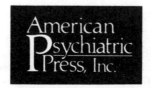

American Psychiatric Press, Inc.

1400 K Street, N.W.
Washington, DC 20005

Cover design by Sam Haltom
Text design by Richard E. Farkas
Typeset by Monotype Composition Co., Inc.
Printed by Semline, Inc.

Library of Congress Cataloging in Publication Data

Schatzberg, Alan F.
  Manual of clinical psychopharmacology.

  Includes index.
  1. Mental illness—Chemotherapy. 2. Psychopharmacology.
3. Psychotropic drugs. I. Cole, Jonathan O. II. Title. [DNLM: 1. Mental Disorders—drug therapy. 2. Psychotropic Drugs—pharmacodynamics. QV 77 S312m]
RC483.S37   1986   616.89′18   86-1929
ISBN 0-88048-036-X (pbk.)

Dedication

To Evelyn M. Stone
without whose encouragement and support
this book would not have been written.

Contents

1 General Principles of Psychopharmacologic Treatment   1

2 Diagnosis and Classification   11

3 Antidepressants   27

4   Antipsychotic Drugs   67

5 | Mood Stabilizers 107

List of Tables

List of Figures

Acknowledgments

Our wives and families deserve special thanks for allowing us the time and effort needed on nights and weekends to prepare and complete this book. Elaine Beroz, Barbara Balse, and Laurin Ericson prepared and revised the manuscript and tables for publication.

This book grows out of our work at McLean Hospital over the past twelve years. Credit is due to Dr. Shervert H. Frazier who recruited us to McLean Hospital as well as to all our colleagues, particularly our residents and staff in the Affective Disease Program. Last, the many patients we have tried to help over the years deserve much thanks. We hope that the next decade will bring even better treatments to ameliorate the suffering of psychiatric patients.

General Principles of Psychopharmacologic Treatment

Psychiatry has experienced a rapid metamorphosis over the past two decades in its methods of treatment. The move from a largely psychoanalytic orientation toward a more biological stance has not only radically changed our basic approaches to patients but also our own professional identities. For most psychiatrists, the transformation has not been easy. Keeping up with the ever-expanding information on biological theories, new laboratory tests, computerization, new medications, and new additional uses for old medications has in itself been a full-time occupation, one which often allows little time or energy to integrate current information into daily practice. Moreover, the proliferation of biological and psychopharmacologic information has occurred so rapidly that the task of integrating biological and psychotherapeutic approaches is made ever more difficult.

Some academics and practitioners would argue that psychopharmacologic approaches have become the essence of psychiatry, whereas others may insist that these drugs merely mask underlying diseases, work against conflict resolution, interfere with therapy, etc. Our impression has been that many, if not most, practitioners have developed more balanced, practical approaches which combine elements of both dynamic psychotherapy and psychopharmacology. In an odd way, academic psychiatry with its sometimes hypertrophied and polarized approaches has lagged *behind* clinical practice. Indeed, intuitively, we believe that psychiatry as a medical subspecialty will eventually incorporate aspects of psychosocial, psychobiological, and psychopharmacologic theories to form a truly "new psychiatry." One major reason for this is that although psychotropic drugs exert profound and beneficial effects on cognition, mood, and behavior, they often do not change the underlying disease process which is frequently highly sensitive to intrapsychic, intrapersonal, and psychosocial stressors. As a rule, beneficial outcomes can only be achieved by simultaneously reducing symptoms and promoting the capacity of the individual to adapt to the exigencies of his or her life. Strikingly, some practitioners of internal medicine have already come to embrace psychosocial principles to help such illnesses as hypertension, juvenile diabetes, ulcer disease, etc. Similarly, psychiatrists who overly embrace psychopharmacology as the be-all and end-all will probably find themselves in the same position as internists who feel prescribing thiazides is a simple solution to hypertensive illness. Conversely, practitioners of psychoanalysis should not expect that approach to "cure" or significantly reduce vegetative symptomatology in endogenously depressed patients. Rather they need to realize the potential benefits of alternative treatments—particularly psychotropic medication.

For practitioners who have not had extensive experience, a transition to a more pharmacologic practice is not without difficulties. A favorable clinical outcome after prescribing a psychotropic drug does reinforce confidence in psychopharmacologic approaches. Practically speaking, favorable outcomes can often be effected more quickly with a psychopharmacologic approach than with psychotherapy, so that confidence in psychopharmacology can be achieved readily.

Although this book is primarily a guide to psychopharmacology, its contents should not lead the reader to conclude that understanding how to select and prescribe psychotropic medications obviates the basic need to comprehensively evaluate and understand psychiatric patients. Our primary purpose is to provide the reader/practitioner with basic and practical information regarding the many classes of psychiatric medications. This book is written as a practical, usable clinical guide to the selection and prescription of appropriate drug therapies for individual patients, drawing on our own *clinical* experience as well as on the scientific literature. It is *not* a series of meticulously documented review papers, so individual statements in the text are not individually referenced. However, each chapter is followed by a list of selected relevant papers and books for readers who wish to go beyond the material presented here.

GENERAL ADVICE

For the less experienced practitioner of psychopharmacology, a number of practical steps can be followed to assist in the development of skills and in the achievement of favorable outcomes.

Generally speaking, we recommend that practitioners concentrate first on one or two drugs per drug class and become fully familiar with how to use them (dosage, side effects, etc.). One's armamentarium of medication can then be widened over time and through further experience. The physician should have available some key resource materials—textbooks on psychopharmacology, *Physicians' Desk Reference (PDR)*, etc. (Some helpful titles are listed on page 267.) These can be supplemented with pharmacology newsletters, which provide useful current information. Moreover, practitioners should be familiar with a number of books

directed at the lay audience that can help supplement information provided to patients (see Suggested Reading List on
page 267). It is also a good idea to identify local psychopharmacologic consultants who can provide second opinions
when needed, such as if patients fail to respond or if they
experience severe side effects.

LEGAL/ETHICAL ISSUES

It seems prudent to discuss briefly a number of legal and
ethical issues that have arisen in psychopharmacology. Since
a comprehensive discussion of all of these is beyond the scope
of this guide, the reader is referred elsewhere for specific
information (see Suggested Reading List).

Informed consent has become an increasingly important
issue in medicine. Standard medical practice has long called
for informing patients of the risk/benefit ratio of various
surgical and medical procedures. More recently, greater
attention has been paid to the question of informed consent;
for psychiatry, however, several key problems quickly arise.
For one, psychiatrists must wrestle with the dilemma of
evaluating the patient's capacity either to understand fully
the benefits and risks of the medication prescribed or to
interpret the provided information in a reflective and beneficial way. Obviously, this issue is particularly pressing in the
psychotic patient, and legal guardianship may be required at
times to effect adequate informed consent. Fortunately, these
patients represent a minority of the average practitioner's
patient population.

The paranoid, but competent, patient presents practical
problems that are best overcome by creating a solid working
relationship. Such patients are less commonly encountered
than are highly anxious, obsessive, or agitated patients who
are prone to adopt a phobic approach to medication. The
practitioner at first glance may view informed consent in

such cases as an insurmountable obstacle. Practically speaking, however, such patients will be anxious even if one does *not* inform them of side effects. Indeed, disclosing the facts often relieves their anxiety. It also connotes a respect for the severity of their illness and the need to mutually assume some risks.

Should the physician inform the patient of every side effect listed in *PDR* or merely highlight the most common ones? Some courts have judged that physicians may be liable if they do not tell the patient of every side effect. Practically speaking, most clinicians do not do so for several reasons, including the time involved and concern of unduly frightening the patient. The latter is particularly relevant when one reflects on the fact that package insert information lists virtually all side effects ever reported in drug trials, even if they were not due to the drug, plus side effects observed only or mainly on similar drugs. Still, we are impressed that patients not only have ready access to copies of *PDR* and consumer guides to medications but also commonly use them. In a sense, these practices begin to obviate the practitioner's perceived dilemma. Physicians need to enter into an open dialogue with all patients regarding the benefits and side effects of medication, even or particularly those patients who are self-taught. Patients who read *PDR* need to be informed of the relative probability of one or another side effect occurring. For example, patients should be made to realize that a dry mouth as the result of a tricyclic antidepressant is to be expected, but agranulocytosis or anaphylaxis is extremely rare. Our experience is that patients are reassured by the physician's belief (and hope) that these side effects will not be encountered. Recent package inserts often include tables comparing side effects on a given drug to those observed on placebo. This places the issues in a much better perspective.

Some physicians routinely hand to patients written materials (often a separate sheet for each medication) that spell out the medication's relative risks. This works well, but only if the practitioner feels comfortable with it and it becomes truly routine in his or her practice.

A particularly difficult problem revolves around the informed consent of risk for developing tardive dyskinesia, an unfortunate side reaction generally due to *long-term* treatment with antipsychotic medication (see Chapter 4). Tardive dyskinesia is a real risk in psychiatric practice. It affects some 14 percent of patients maintained on neuroleptic medication for three or more years and may be more common in patients with affective disorders than in those with schizophrenia. Thus, practitioners need to be particularly conservative in administering neuroleptics to patients who do not demonstrate frequent or chronic psychotic episodes. However, since chronic psychotic disorders do unfortunately exist, even prudent practice cannot eliminate the risk for tardive dyskinesia.

What should the physician tell the patient about tardive dyskinesia and when? Here a variety of approaches have been developed. One is to inform the patient and/or the family of the risk of tardive dyskinesia before prescribing neuroleptics. This may be too anxiety provoking and impractical, particularly for the acutely psychotic patient, since tardive dyskinesia generally is a long-term side effect and there is a pressing need to help compensate the patient quickly. Another approach is to broach the subject of the risk of tardive dyskinesia after approximately four to six weeks of treatment, before embarking on long-term or maintenance therapy. This seems more prudent to us.

Should one obtain written verification of informed consent? Here, too, different approaches have emerged. Some institutions and practitioners have adopted formal written informed consent. Others have adopted traditional verbal informed consent procedures and written documentation of the interchange in the patient's record. Still others have routinely provided the patient with additional written information regarding risks of tardive dyskinesia or other side effects (beyond *PDR*) but have not asked the patient to provide written informed consent. Each of these approaches has its advantages and its proponents. Currently, we recommend that practitioners and institutions adopt some formal documented disclosure of the risk of tardive dyskinesia and that they combine this with conservative administration of neuroleptics (both in terms of time and dosage) and a mutually cooperative undertaking of monitoring patients for the emergence of dyskinetic movements.

In the past decade, physicians have been increasingly faced with the dilemma of prescribing standard drugs for indications that have not been approved by the U.S. Food and Drug Administration (FDA) or at doses that are higher than those recommended in *PDR*. In some instances, drugs can be misprescribed, and this can obviously be dangerous. In many others, considerable clinical or research data have emerged pointing to potentially great benefits to many patients, but package insert information may not have been changed because of economic or regulatory factors. For example, imipramine today is commonly prescribed to both outpatients and inpatients at doses of 300 mg/day. Still, the package insert states that outpatients should not receive more than 225 mg/day. In part, this reflects the fact that approved dosage regimens were determined on the basis of data generated many years ago when a greater proportion of seriously depressed patients were treated as inpatients and before the application of plasma levels (see Chapter 3). It is unlikely that the package insert will be changed. Additional studies to further document the efficacy and safety of higher dosages would be too costly for drug manufacturers, who can no longer hope to recoup the costs of such study since the patent for the drug may have long since expired. One pharmaceutical manufacturer several years ago applied for and was granted FDA approval to raise the maximum daily dose of its nortriptyline compound (Pamelor) from 100 to

150 mg/day. A manufacturer of an identical nortriptyline compound—Aventyl—did not, and this product enjoys only a 100 mg maximum daily dose. Thus, we have on the U.S. market two identical nortriptylines with different maximum daily doses.

Examples of so-called nonapproved uses include the use of imipramine and phenelzine for patients with agoraphobia or panic disorder or that of carbamazepine in manic-depressive illness. There is a growing body of data that these drugs are effective, but market conditions and regulatory guidelines may result in some, or even all, of these drugs not being granted official new indications. Is the practitioner at legal risk in prescribing these drugs? Generally, the American Medical Association and FDA have taken the position that the use of any marketed drug for "nonapproved" indications or at higher dosages for individual patients is within the purview of the clinician. *PDR* is not an official textbook of medical practice but rather a compendium of drug information for marketing purposes. It sets limitations on what pharmaceutical companies can claim for their products. Malpractice is based on failure to practice within community norms. Still, many clinicians will not easily accept the potential risk of being sued—even if such a suit may have little merit— by a patient who experiences an untoward reaction to a standard drug used for a "nonapproved" indication or to a dose of drug that is higher than the recommended maximum dose.

What are the solutions? Until various forces (both patients and physicians) come to the fore to effect a change in the system for widening indications or for maximum doses, each clinician must decide whether he or she wishes to assume the risk. However, while clinicians may attempt to opt for a conservative approach, they will at some point encounter patients who will require alternative treatments. One possible aid may be to acquire outside consultation from more expert psychopharmacologists or from other practitioners in the community. Another is to explain the scope of the problem to patients, providing them with available published reports on positive benefits, and documenting this in their records. Some physicians will ask for written documentation that the patient has been informed. In the end, there are no simple solutions, and the physician will at some point be faced with this problem.

In this book, we have attempted to provide practical information regarding many different psychotropic drugs. Information regarding dosages is for adult patients (ages 18-60 years) unless otherwise noted. We have included information derived from our reading of the psychiatric literature as well as from our own clinical practice. We have attempted to indicate, wherever possible, those uses that officially have not been approved by the FDA for marketing purposes, but we have also attempted to provide the readers with sufficient data so that they can decide whether or how they may wish to prescribe specific drugs. In so doing, we are not endorsing their use but are realistically attempting to place a drug in its proper perspective. We believe "real-world" psychiatric practice dictates that we provide the practitioner with information based on either the scientific literature or on common clinical use, even though a drug's indications may yet not have been changed or—perhaps because of economic reasons—may never be changed.

Bibliography

Applebaum PS: Legal and ethical aspects of psychopharmacologic practice, in Clinical Psychopharmacology, 2nd ed. Edited by Bernstein JC. Boston, Wright PSG, 1984

Erickson SH, Bergman JJ, Schneeweiss R, et al: The use of drugs for unlabeled indications. JAMA 243:1543–1546, 1980

The FDA Does Not Approve Uses of Drugs [editorial]. JAMA 252:1054–1055, 1984

Nonapproved uses of FDA-approved drugs. JAMA 211:1705, 1970

Use of approved drugs for unlabeled indications. FDA Drug Bull, April 1982

Use of drug for unapproved indications: your legal responsibility. FDA Drug Bull, October 1972

Diagnosis and Classification

2

In recent years psychiatry has paid increasing attention to diagnosis and classification, reaching a peak with the publication of the *Diagnostic and Statistical Manual of Mental Disorders,* Third Edition (*DSM-III*). Much of this attention has been sparked by advances in the biology and treatment of various psychiatric disorders, making precise diagnosis ever more important. For example, the response of many patients diagnosed with bipolar (manic-depressive) illness to lithium carbonate has fostered the adoption of rigorous efforts to discriminate between manic-depressive illness and schizophrenia, resulting in both a change of diagnosis of many patients and subsequent alterations in their treatment.

Approaches to psychopharmacologic treatment are often based on trying to match a given treatment or a combination of treatments with a specific diagnosis. Although this approach represents the ideal, it is only effective in approximately 60 percent of patients since

a. many patients have a disorder that is not easily classified;

11

b. some patients with a seemingly classic disorder may not respond to a traditional drug;

c. increasingly, various drugs have been shown to exert wider actions than their drug class eponym (e.g., anticonvulsants) suggests.

Thus, the clinician must combine the "ideal" paradigm with a more flexible approach—one that attempts to match a given treatment with various clusters of symptoms rather than with an overall syndrome. The danger of this approach, however, is that—if carried too far—it can result in unhealthy polypharmacy. Obviously, the clinician must attempt to develop a general strategy for matching a range of specific treatments to patients with particular diagnoses or symptoms.

A sound general philosophy is to ascertain whether patients meet symptom criteria for a disorder (e.g., major depression with melancholia) that is generally thought to commonly respond to a given class of drug or treatment (e.g., tricyclic antidepressants) and then to prescribe classic representatives of the given drug class (e.g., imipramine). This can later be followed by a shift to less traditional medications if initial trials do not prove to be effective. Such an approach is sound overall; however, clinicians must be aware that diagnostic classifications have inherent limitations that can be misleading. For example, it is our impression that many patients diagnosed with *DSM-III* major depression do not respond to antidepressant drugs, often requiring some form of psychotherapy (e.g., interpersonal psychotherapy, cognitive therapy, etc.). In part we believe this is due to the limited number and type of symptoms that are required for a disorder to be diagnosed as major depression. Indeed, although major depression is commonly mistaken as representing an endogenous type of depressive illness, in fact—historically and practically speaking—endogenous depression (which is classically believed to respond to tricyclic antidepressants) is only a subtype of major depression.

Although comprehensive discussion of psychiatric classification is beyond the scope of this monograph, it is useful to review *DSM-III* diagnosis and the prevalence of major categories of adult psychiatric disorders and to highlight which types of psychopharmacologic agents often prove most beneficial in each. Prevalence rates provided in this chapter are based primarily on recent reports from the Epidemiologic Catchment Area Program. Table 2-A summarizes *DSM-III* disorders described in this chapter. At the time of publication a revision of *DSM-III* criteria (*DSM-III-R*) had been proposed, but because it is still under review, it is not considered in this chapter.

AFFECTIVE DISORDERS

Affective disorders by definition are pathological mood states. Broadly speaking, on the basis of severity these disorders are divided into "major affective" and "other specific" subcategories. These are then further broken down along a bipolar versus unipolar dimension.

Major Affective Disorder

To be diagnosed as having a *bipolar disorder* (manic-depressive illness), the patient must currently meet criteria for hypomania or mania or must have had a prior episode that met criteria for either of these syndromes. The current episode is further categorized according to whether the patient is manic, depressed, or is experiencing a mixed affect state.

Criteria for mania include at least three of seven symptoms: increase in activity, increased speaking, flight of ideas, inflated self-esteem, decreased need for sleep, distractibility, and overinvolvement in and unawareness of high-risk activities (e.g., spending sprees, reckless driving, etc.). Since only a limited number of symptoms need be present and for only a relatively brief period (one week), some investigators and

Table 2-A. *DSM-III* Diagnoses Addressed

I. *Affective Disorders*
  A. Major affective
    1. Bipolar Disorder
    2. Major Depression
  B. Other specific
    1. Cyclothymic
    2. Dysthymic (depressive neurosis)
II. *Schizophrenic Disorders*
III. *Psychotic Disorders Not Elsewhere Classified*
  A. Schizophreniform
  B. Schizoaffective
IV. *Anxiety Disorders*
  A. Phobias
    1. Simple
    2. Social
    3. Agoraphobia with or without panic attacks
  B. Anxiety States
    1. Panic
    2. Generalized anxiety
    3. Obsessive-compulsive
  C. Post-Traumatic Stress
V. *Somatoform Disorders*
  A. Psychogenic pain
VI. *Personality Disorder*
  A. Borderline
  B. Paranoid
  C. Antisocial
VII. *Substance Use Disorders*
  A. Alcohol abuse
  B. Alcohol dependence
  C. Non-alcohol substance abuse*
  D. Non-alcohol substance dependence*
VIII. *Disorders of Childhood and Adolescence*
  A. Bulimia
  B. Attention deficit disorder

* Includes abuse/dependence involving various agents.

clinicians have argued that the criteria are too broad. The prevalence of mania in the general population is approximately 1 percent.

The classic psychopharmacologic treatment approach for overall mood stabilization of this disorder involves lithium carbonate or lithium citrate; recently, carbamazepine, valproic acid, and clonazepam have also been shown to have mood-stabilizing effects, most prominently in acute mania (see Chapter 5). Treatment of acute hypomania or mania includes the mood-stabilizing drugs noted above as well as antipsychotic, neuroleptic agents and sedative hypnotics for sleep. Treatment of bipolar depression often requires combining lithium with treatments used for major depression (see below).

As described above, the major strides made toward a wider redefinition of bipolar manic states have undoubtedly resulted in more patients receiving lithium carbonate. The potential benefit to many patients in this broadening of diagnoses must be weighed against a procrustean tendency to overdiagnose the disorder in order to justify lithium treatment. Not uncommonly, one sees patients who have a chronic disorder that was once termed schizophrenia but has now been rediagnosed as either a bipolar manic-depressive or schizoaffective illness. Unfortunately, many such patients do not respond to lithium, pointing to certain inherent limitations in overbroadening this category.

Major depression is by definition a *unipolar disorder*. Six-month and lifetime prevalence rates are 2-3 percent and 3-6 percent, respectively, and women are more commonly affected than men. Criteria for major depression consist of a variety of signs and symptoms, including appetite disturbance, sleep disturbance, psychomotor retardation or agitation, suicidality, decreased interest in life, and guilt. Obviously, many of these symptoms are those that European and American investigators have used to describe "endogenous depression." Unfortunately, a patient may meet criteria for major depression without demonstrating much in the way of endogenous symptoms since only four symptoms are required. Moreover, only two weeks duration of symptoms are needed to meet criteria.

A subtype of major depression ("with melancholia") more

closely resembles "endogenous depression." Criteria for this subtype include distinct loss of pleasure in activities, lack of reactivity to pleasurable stimuli, and three of the following: lowering of mood, diurnal variation, marked psychomotor retardation, early morning awakening, significant weight loss, and excessive guilt. It is not yet clear whether major depression with melancholia will fully approximate endogenous depression, since similarly brief time constraints are applied as they are in major depression. Further research will hopefully lead to even better phenomenologic definition of this disorder.

An important subtype of major depression—"major depression with psychotic features"—by definition involves delusional thinking as evidenced by guilty or nihilistic delusions, hallucinations, and even communicative incompetence. This specific disorder represents some 6-15 percent of all major depressions.

Primary treatments for major depression include tricyclic antidepressants (TCAs), monoamine oxidase inhibitors (MAOIs), electroconvulsive therapy (ECT), trazodone, and bupropion. Secondary treatments are lithium carbonate and the triazolobenzodiazepine, alprazolam. Major depression with psychotic features often does poorly with tricyclics alone; rather it may require a combination of tricyclics and phenothiazines or ECT.

Other Specific Affective Disorders

Cyclothymic disorder is a more chronic and less severe illness than bipolar disorder. A two-year course with repeated episodes of mild mood cycles is required to meet criteria for this disorder. Many investigators claim that lithium carbonate is of benefit to some patients with this disorder.

Dysthymic disorder (depressive neurosis) is a more chronic condition whose symptoms by definition are not severe enough to meet criteria for major depression. In addition, a number of the symptom criteria are not endogenous in nature, e.g., anxiety, irritability, and obsessionality. Its six-month and lifetime prevalences are approximately 2-4 percent. There is little evidence that antidepressants are truly effective in this condition; however, if the condition is severe enough, they may prove helpful. Probably related to dysthymic disorder (but not identical with it) is "atypical depression," a nonendogenous depressive illness with pronounced anxiety, for which English psychiatrists have long advocated MAOIs.

SCHIZOPHRENIC DISORDERS

Schizophrenic disorders are disorders of cognition and thinking—in contrast to disorders of mood. These syndromes are heterogeneous with multiple subtypes described in *DSM-III*. Of particular importance in these conditions are delusions (often persecutory in nature), hallucinations (primarily auditory), and/or thought disorder or disruption in thinking. Further, the illness' course is chronic (at least six months) and often deteriorating, and the patient commonly shows social isolation and withdrawal. Six-month and lifetime prevalence rates of schizophrenic disorders are 1-2 percent. Primary treatments are the neuroleptic antipsychotics, which include—for example—phenothiazines, butyrophenones, and thioxanthenes. Some investigators have reported limited benefit with lithium, and the efficacy of tricyclics for some anergic/depressed schizophrenics has also been demonstrated, interestingly, with a relatively low incidence of worsening of psychosis.

Schizophreniform and schizoaffective disorders are subsumed under "psychotic disorders not elsewhere classified." Schizophreniform disorders differ from schizophrenia only in duration of illness—lasting from two weeks to six months. This is a rarer disorder with six-month and lifetime prevalence rates varying between 0.1-0.3 percent. Acute treatment for this condition generally involves neuroleptics. Schizoaffective disorder is used when the history is not clear enough to allow

for a more precise diagnosis (e.g., bipolar disorder, schizophrenia, etc.). For example, some patients with an episodic
illness with both affective and schizophrenic features and
with residual evidence of psychosis when in "remission" may
receive this diagnosis. Such patients often receive the most
complex drug regimens in a valiant effort to control a mix
of affective, schizophrenic, and even anxiety symptoms.

ANXIETY DISORDERS

The *DSM-III* classification of anxiety disorders is radically
different from its *DSM-II* predecessor; however, efforts are
already underway to reorganize this section of *DSM-III*.
Anxiety in *DSM-III* is divided into two main categories:
phobias and anxiety states. Phobias are subdivided into simple
(e.g., animals, storms, etc.), social (interpersonal situations,
public speaking, etc.), and agoraphobia (fear of open spaces
or of being alone) with or without panic attacks. The anxiety
states are divided into generalized anxiety disorder, panic
disorder, post-traumatic stress disorder, and obsessive-compulsive disorder.

Whereas considerable progress in classifying anxiety is
reflected in *DSM-III*, a great deal of confusion and debate
still remains. This is particularly evident in the questions of
how and where to subdivide the group of disorders included
under agoraphobia, agoraphobia with panic attacks, panic
disorder, and generalized anxiety disorder.

Phobic Disorders

The *simple phobias* include encapsulated fears of specific
stimuli (heights, animals, closed spaces, etc.). Animal phobias
are almost exclusively found in females and generally begin
in childhood. The six-month and lifetime prevalence rates of
simple phobias are extremely high—approximately 5 and 10
percent, respectively. The conditions are generally treated
with behavior therapy.

Social phobias involve intense and undue fears of interpersonal interactions, urinating in public bathrooms, etc. They occur in both sexes and begin in early adulthood.

Agoraphobia—the fear of being alone or in open spaces (e.g., supermarkets or shopping malls)—has attracted increasing attention in recent years, as particularly seen in numerous psychopharmacologic and psychotherapeutic studies on agoraphobia with panic attacks, a *DSM-III* subtype of agoraphobia. Agoraphobia is far more common in women than men, and the mean age of onset is the late 20s. The lifetime prevalence rate of agoraphobia is approximately 4 percent. The disorder can be disabling since patients may markedly constrict their daily activities. The phobic aspects may be treated via behavioral therapy or psychotherapy. Acute symptomatic relief may be best effected by using benzodiazepines. Overall, however, agoraphobia with panic attacks is highly responsive to alprazolam, imipramine, and phenelzine.

Anxiety States

Panic disorder is characterized by at least three episodes of panic—acute, almost incapacitating anxiety—in a three-week period. These attacks are characterized by dyspnea, chest discomfort, palpitations, lightheadedness, sense of dread, hot and cold flashes, sweating, faintness, etc. If they are associated with agoraphobia, a diagnosis of agoraphobia with panic is made. The six-month and lifetime prevalence rates of panic disorder are approximately 0.6 and 1.5 percent, respectively, and the disorder is more common in women than men. There has been considerable debate whether there is a meaningful difference between panic and agoraphobia with panic since some investigators have posited that agoraphobia is a form of end-stage avoidance behavior to defend against possible panic attacks. Indeed, they have even argued that generalized anxiety disorder is an end-stage generalization of earlier panic symptoms, so-called endogenous anxiety.

Since patients having agoraphobia with panic respond to alprazolam, imipramine, and phenelzine, it is generally presumed that patients with panic disorder will respond similarly.

Generalized anxiety disorder is characterized by persistent anxiety of at least one month. Symptoms include motor tension—shakiness, tension, trembling, etc; autonomic hyperactivity—sweating, heart pounding, cold hands, etc.; apprehensive expectation—anxiety, worry, fear, etc.; and vigilance and scanning—difficulty in concentrating, insomnia, irritability, etc. The disorder is more common in women than men, and prevalence rates range between 2 and 6 percent. A variety of drug classes may be effective in generalized anxiety disorder, including benzodiazepines, barbiturates, antihistamines, phenothiazines, and meprobamate. However, of these medications, benzodiazepines are overwhelmingly the most commonly prescribed. Recently, tricyclic antidepressants have also been shown to be effective in treating this disorder.

Obsessive-compulsive disorder is characterized by obsessions and compulsions producing significant distress. Obsessions are recurrent, persistent ideas and thoughts that are ego-dystonic. Compulsions are defined as "repetitive and seemingly purposeful behaviors performed according to rules or in a stereotyped fashion." Also, more common in women than men, six-month and lifetime prevalence rates are 1.5 and 3.0 percent, respectively. Often, patients with pronounced obsessive-compulsive symptoms are at closer inspection found to meet criteria for major depression. Preliminary studies suggest that clomipramine, a tricyclic antidepressant, may be particularly effective in this condition. Other tricyclics and MAOIs have been found, in limited studies, to be somewhat effective.

Post-traumatic stress disorder has come under increased scrutiny since the Vietnam War. The disorder is characterized by the existence of a recognizable stressor that would be inferred to potentially evoke distress in most individuals. Previous trauma is reexperienced via recurrent recollections or dreams of the event or a sudden sense that the event was recurring. Often, these patients demonstrate decreased responsiveness or involvement with the external world. Common symptoms include startle responses, memory or concentration problems, sleep disturbance, guilt about surviving, avoidance of stimuli which mimic or simulate the event, and recrudescence of symptoms upon exposure of stimuli. Although the disorder has achieved wide popular interest because of the political aspects of the war in Vietnam, similar disorders have long been known in the literature, such as traumatic war neurosis in World War II pilots. The prevalence of the disorder is unclear. Also, psychopharmacologic treatment has not been well studied but a number of preliminary open studies suggest that phenelzine (an MAOI) and alprazolam may be effective.

SOMATOFORM DISORDERS

Somatoform disorders represent a class of disorders that involve physical complaints that are without objective medical basis. Four major illnesses in this group are somatization disorder, conversion disorder, psychogenic pain disorder, and hypochondriasis. The prevalence rate of this group of disorders is approximately 0.1 percent, and women predominate. Psychogenic pain disorder has been reported to respond to antidepressant therapy. The other disorders have not been shown to be particularly responsive to psychopharmacologic therapy.

PERSONALITY DISORDERS

In *DSM-III,* personality disorder diagnoses are made under Axis II. Generally, these disorders have not been found to respond to psychopharmacologic treatment; however, medication may reduce certain symptoms. Three personality disorders are of particular note for this manual: borderline personality disorder, paranoid personality disorder, and antisocial personality disorder.

Borderline personality disorder, which has attracted great interest and study in recent years, is characterized by impulsivity; unstable and intense interpersonal relationships; inappropriate, intense anger; identity disturbances; affective instability; self-destructive physical acts; and a chronic sense of emptiness. This disorder (or variants thereof) may respond to lithium carbonate (emotionally unstable character), phenelzine (hysteroid dysphoria), low dosages of thioridazine or thiothixene, and carbamazepine ("wrist slashers").

Paranoid personality disorder is characterized by pervasive unwarranted suspiciousness, hypersensitivity, and restricted affectivity. By definition, the paranoia is not due to schizophrenia or paranoid disorder. Although the somatic treatment of paranoid personality has not been well studied, trials of phenothiazines or lithium carbonate may prove useful in this disorder.

Antisocial personality disorder is characterized by chronic antisocial behavior, with onset before age 15. This disorder is far more common in men than in women. Six-month and lifetime prevalence rates for the disorder are approximately 0.6 and 2.0 percent, respectively.

Substance Use Disorders

Two major classes of substance abuse or dependence (alcohol and drugs) have been emphasized in *DSM-III.* Abuse reflects pathologic use of a substance or impairment in social and occupational performance secondary to substance use. Dependence includes psychological need for continuing a substance as well as abuse of, tolerance to, or withdrawal from the particular substance. The prevalence of substance use disorders is unfortunately high in this country. Six-month and lifetime prevalence rates for alcohol dependence abuse are approximately 5 and 14 percent, respectively. Alcohol abuse dependence is five times more common in men than in women; drug abuse/dependence is somewhat less common with six-month and lifetime prevalence rates of 2 and 5 percent, respectively. These disorders are only slightly more common in men than in women. In disorders involving substance use or abuse, pharmacologic treatment is generally aimed at ameliorating symptoms of withdrawal or at promoting abstinence either by producing physical discomfort in the face of intoxication (e.g., disulfiram for alcohol abuse) or by blocking drug-induced euphoria (e.g., methadone or naltrexone). When the substance has been abused in the context of another disorder (such as major depression) treatment of the underlying disorder is warranted (such as with a tricyclic antidepressant).

"CHILDHOOD AND ADOLESCENT" DISORDERS

Two disorders that in *DSM-III* are subsumed under disorders of onset in childhood or adolescence deserve some mention. Bulimia, characterized by intense eating binges, occurs in both adolescents and adults and has been thought by some investigators to be related to depression or affective disease. While there is some debate as to the nature of the possible relationship, it is clear that many bulimic patients respond to treatment with tricyclic antidepressants or monoamine oxidase inhibitors. Some bulimics also respond to behavior therapy. The other syndrome—attention deficit disorder—is characterized by hyperactivity and poor attention span. Classically, it has its onset in childhood, but an adult form almost certainly exists (usually in patients who were hyperactive as children). The disorder responds well to stimulants and may also respond to tricyclic antidepressants and perhaps to monoamine oxidase inhibitors as well.

In summary, accurate diagnosis and classification provide clues for developing psychopharmacologic strategies. How-

Table 2-B. Common and Possible Uses of Classes of Psychotropic Medications

Antidepressant drugs (Including probably alprazolam)	Major depressive disorders Agoraphobia with panic Bipolar disorders, depressed (with lithium) ? Generalized anxiety disorder ? Depression as a symptom in other primary disorders ? Psychogenic pain disorder Bulimia
Antipsychotic drugs	Schizophrenic disorder Schizophreniform disorder Schizoaffective disorder Bipolar disorder, manic phase Agitated organic disorders ? Treatment-resistant major depression ? Borderline personality disorder
Antianxiety drugs	Generalized anxiety disorder Anxiety symptoms in other psychiatric disorders Akathisia Detoxification of alcohol dependence disorder
Stimulants	Adult attentional deficit disorder ? Treatment-resistant depressive disorders
Lithium carbonate	Bipolar disorder Major depression (single episode or recurrent) Schizoaffective disorder ? Impulse disorders ? Cyclothymic disorder
Antiseizure drugs	Bipolar disorder Psychosis of temporal lobe epilepsy ? Major depression, particularly atypical or treatment-resistant subtype
Hypnotics	Sleep disturbance of mania, depression, anxiety, or other disorders

? indicates possible uses.

ever, the clinician should not expect to find 1:1 correlations between the types of patients encountered in practice and the classic prototypes in the literature. This may prove particularly important when one is following a patient over many years. In such a case, a flexible approach needs to be developed, one which includes routine and rather regular reassessment of the patient's condition, a need for changes in medication, etc. Table 2-B illustrates the complex interdigitation of drug classes and psychiatric disorders. These issues are discussed in more detail in the following chapters.

Bibliography

American Psychiatric Association: Diagnostic and Statistical Manual of Mental Disorders, 3rd ed. Washington, DC, American Psychiatric Association, 1980

Boyd JH, Burke JD, Gruenberg E: Exclusion criteria of DSM-III: a study of co-occurrence of hierarchy-free syndromes. Arch Gen Psychiatry 41:983–989, 1984

Marks I, Lader M: Anxiety states (anxiety neurosis): a review. J Nerv Ment Dis 156:3–18, 1973

Myers JK, Weissman MM, Tischler GL, et al: Six-month prevalence of psychiatric disorders in three communities. Arch Gen Psychiatry 41:959–967, 1984

Pope HG, Lipinski JF: Diagnosis in schizophrenia and manic-depressive illness: a reassessment of the specificity of "schizophrenic" symptoms in the light of current research. Arch Gen Psychiatry 35:811–828, 1978

Robins LN, Helzer JE, Weissman MM, et al: Lifetime prevalence of specific psychiatric disorders in three sites. Arch Gen Psychiatry 41:949–958, 1984

Schatzberg AF: Classification of affective disorders, in The Brain, Biochemistry, and Behavior (Proceedings of the Sixth Arnold O. Beckman Conference in Clinical Chemistry). Edited by Habig RL. Washington, DC, American Association for Clinical Chemistry, 1984

Sheehan DV, Sheehan KH: The classification of anxiety and hysterical states, part I: historical review and empirical delineation. J Clin Psychopharmacol 2:235–244, 1982

Sheehan DV, Sheehan KH: The classification of anxiety and hysterical states, part II: towards a more heuristic classification. J Clin Psychopharmacol 2:386–393, 1982

Antidepressants

3

The class of drugs labelled antidepressants has widened dramatically in the past five years with the introduction of several new forms within this class. Classic antidepressants include the tricyclic antidepressants (TCAs) and related tetracyclics as well as the monoamine oxidase inhibitors (MAOIs). The newer agents (e.g., trazodone, nomifensine, bupropion, and fluoxetine) differ in structure from the classic medications and offer some advantages in terms of alternative biological actions and side-effect profiles although, overall, they are probably no more effective than previous pharmacologic agents. For patients who cannot tolerate or have not responded to the more traditional agents, these newer medications prove useful. For the clinician, learning to use them represents a great challenge, particularly when one considers the task of trying to catch up with the ever-expanding and increasingly more complicated uses of traditional antidepressant medications.

HISTORY

Classic antidepressants were originally discovered serendipitously. In the early 1950s, investigators noted that tuberculosis patients showed prolonged elevation of mood when treated with iproniazid, an MAOI thought to be an antituberculosis agent. This MAOI proved ineffective for tuberculosis, but its impact on mood led to some of the earliest double-blind studies in psychopharmacology, which demonstrated that MAOIs were effective antidepressant agents. The biologic and pharmacologic observations that MAOIs were antidepressants, and that monoamine oxidase degraded norepinephrine and serotonin, became cornerstones of the so-called biogenic amine theories of depression. Iproniazid, however, although available in Great Britain, was taken off the U.S. market some time ago because of fear that it caused hepatic necrosis. For many years the use of other MAOIs declined partly because of the introduction of tricyclic antidepressants, and partly because of the occurrence in patients of significant hypertensive crises.

Tricyclic antidepressants were also discovered serendipitously. The first reports on tricyclic efficacy in depression came from Professor Kuhn in Switzerland, who astutely noted that a three-ringed compound, imipramine, which was being investigated as a treatment for schizophrenia, appeared to elevate mood even though it did not relieve psychosis. The drug was similar in structure to the phenothiazines but a simple substitution of nitrogen for sulfur in the central ring appeared to confer unique psychopharmacologic antidepressant properties.

Two of the newer antidepressants with a four-ringed structure, maprotiline and amoxapine, share similar biochemical effects with the more traditional tricyclics. This is not unexpected, since many antidepressant compounds were developed based on their having similar activity in certain animal models to those of prototypic tricyclic antidepressants, leading some to call them "me too" drugs. However, there are both subtle and pronounced differences between many of the so-called me too drugs. More recently, two new compounds—trazodone and bupropion—with rather unique biological properties have been introduced to the U.S. market. These, along with a host of investigational drugs developed using alternative animal screening, truly represent the second generation of antidepressant drugs.

TRICYCLIC ANTIDEPRESSANTS AND RELATED COMPOUNDS

Indications

The principal "FDA-approved for marketing" indication for tricyclics and related compounds is the treatment of depression—both endogenous and nonendogenous. Other "approved for marketing" indications include anxiety (doxepin) and childhood enuresis (imipramine as an adjunctive treatment). "Nonapproved" but common uses include headache (most commonly amitriptyline, imipramine, and doxepin), agoraphobia with panic attacks (imipramine particularly), chronic pain syndromes (doxepin and maprotiline most frequently), and bulimia (imipramine and desipramine). More recently, imipramine has been reported effective in generalized anxiety disorder, and trimipramine and doxepin may be effective in treating peptic ulcers. The investigational TCA clomipramine may have potent anti-obsessive-compulsive effects. Obviously, these drugs exert rather wide pharmacologic effects, which account for their potentially broad range of actions. (For further discussion of the use of tricyclic antidepressants in anxiety disorders, see the section on antidepressants in Chapter 6.)

There are currently seven tricyclic and two tetracyclic antidepressants on the U.S. market. Their trade and generic names are listed in Table 3-A. The original patents have

Table 3-A. Tricyclic and Tetracyclic Antidepressants

Generic Name	Brand Names	Tablets and Capsules	Oral Concentrate	Parenteral	Therapeutic Dosage Range (mg/day)*
Tricyclics					
amitriptyline	Elavil, Endep Generic	10/25/50/75/100/150 mg	None	10 mg/ml in 10 ml vials	150–300
desipramine	Norpramin Pertofrane	Tablets: 10/25/50/75/100/ 150 mg Capsules: 25/50 mg	None	None	150–300
doxepin	Sinequan Adapin	Capsules: 10/25/50/75/100/ 150 mg	10 mg/ml in 120 ml bottles	None	150–300
imipramine	Tofranil, Janimine, Sk-Pramine Generic	Tablets: 10/25/50 mg	None	25 mg in 2 ml vials	150–300
imipramine pamoate	Tofranil PM (sustained release)	Capsules: 75/100/125/150 mg	None	25 mg in 2 ml vials	150–300
nortriptyline	Pamelor Aventyl	Capsules: 10/25/75 mg	10 mg/5 ml in 16 oz bottles	None	50–150
protriptyline	Vivactil	Tablets: 5/10 mg	None	None	15–60
trimipramine	Surmontil	Capsules: 25/50/100 mg	None	None	150–300
Tetracyclics					
amoxapine	Asendin	Tablets: 25/50/100/150 mg	None	None	150–450
maprotiline	Ludiomil	Tablets: 25/50/75 mg	None	None	150–200

* These dosage ranges are approximate. Many patients will respond at relatively low dosages (even below ranges given above); others may require higher dosages.

expired on several of them, for which generic preparations are now available. In the United States, generic compounds have not been without their controversy. Although they offer a savings for the consumer, some clinicians wonder about their pharmacologic equivalence. One difficulty stems from the FDA definition of bioequivalence, which relies heavily on the demonstration that an identical dosage of a generic preparation produces blood levels comparable to those produced by the original compound. Even with approved generics, some studies have suggested that they are not truly equivalent to standard brands. Moreover, the regulations do not require that pharmaceutical companies prove that their generics enjoy equivalence in clinical or biological potency. This area requires close scrutiny by both clinicians and investigators.

Structures

The chemical structures of tricyclics and related compounds are remarkably similar (Figure 3-1). Desipramine and nortriptyline are demethylated metabolites of imipramine and amitriptyline, respectively. Amoxapine is a derivative of the antipsychotic loxapine and has an additional fourth ring off a side chain. Maprotiline is a four-ring compound, the fourth ring arising perpendicular to the traditional three rings. Its side chain is identical to that of desipramine.

Biochemical Effects

The biochemical effects of these tricyclic and tetracyclic antidepressants are quite similar. Initially, particular emphasis was placed on their relative effects in blocking the reuptake of norepinephrine or serotonin. These differences came to underlie various theories on the biology of depression—particularly the low norepinephrine versus low serotonin hypotheses. In recent years, theories have become more

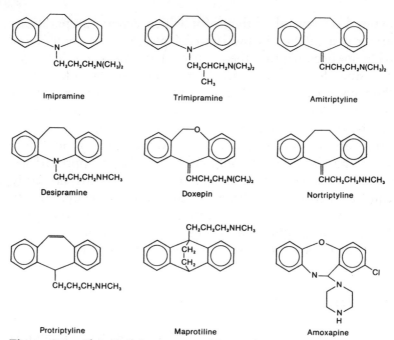

Figure 3-1. Chemical Structures of Tricyclic and Related Antidepressants

complex as the pharmacologic effects of these drugs have been shown to go beyond their mere immediate reuptake blocking effects to include longer term secondary effects on pre- and postsynaptic receptors, as well as on other neurotransmitter systems. The latter effects may account for differences among the various drugs in both their range of efficacy as well as their side effects. At one time, the relative norepinephrine versus serotonin reuptake blocking effects were used to explain the relative sedative (serotonin) versus activating (norepinephrine) properties of these drugs. More recently, sedation, which early on was ascribed to serotoninergic and anticholinergic effects, has in part been ascribed to tricyclics' antihistaminic (H_1 receptor) actions. Anticholinergic effects include dry mouth, constipation, urinary hes-

Table 3-B. Relative Biochemical Effects of Tricyclic and Tetracyclic Drugs

Drug	NE	5-HT	ACH	H_1	H_2
amitriptyline	+	+ +	+ + +	+ +	+ +
desipramine	+ + +	±	+	0	0
doxepin	+	±	+ +	+ + +	+
imipramine	+ +	+	+ +	±	±
nortriptyline	+ +	±	+	±	±
protriptyline	+ + +	±	+ + +	0	0
trimipramine	±	±	+ +	+ +	?
amoxapine	+ +	+	+	?	?
maprotiline	+ + +	0	+	?	?

Note: Biochemical effects include norepinephrine (NE) and serotonin (5-HT) reuptake blocking and binding activity on acetylcholine (ACH) and histamine 1 and 2 (H_1 and H_2) receptors.

itance, blurred vision, and confusion. The H_2 receptor blocking effects may play a role in these drugs, producing weight gain and promoting healing of peptic ulcers.

The relative norepinephrine versus serotonin reuptake blocking effects of these agents are summarized in Table 3-B, as are their relative effects on acetylcholine and H_1 and H_2 receptors. These potencies represent best estimates based on receptor-binding and clinical studies. Variations in biological effects may serve as a guide to drug selection. Table 3-C indicates the types of side effects seen with these compounds.

Dosage Regimen

Having evaluated a depressed patient, the clinician must determine whether TCAs appear to be an appropriate treatment. We subscribe to the approach of using a TCA first in the treatment of endogenous or major depression. Which TCA to use is somewhat a matter of personal preference. There is really considerable overlap among these various drugs, although some are a bit more stimulating (desipramine and protriptyline) and others are more sedating (amitriptyline

Table 3-C. Common or Troublesome Side Effects of Tricyclic and Tetracyclic Drugs

---

I. *Anticholinergic*
   Dry mouth and nasal passages, constipation, urinary hesitance, esophageal reflux
II. *Autonomic*
   Orthostatic hypotension, palpitations, intracardiac conduction slowing, increased sweating, increased blood pressure, tremor
III. *Allergic*
   Skin rashes (maprotiline particularly)
IV. *Central Nervous System*
   Stimulation, sedation, delirium, myoclonic twitches (generally at high dosages), nausea, speech blockage, seizures (particularly with high dosages of maprotiline), and extrapyramidal symptoms (amoxapine)
V. *Other*
   Weight gain and impotence

---

and doxepin). One of us (A.F.S.) tends to start with imipramine, the oldest of these drugs; J.O.C. tends to use imipramine when more sedation is required and desipramine where sedation is potentially a problem. Neither of us employs amitriptyline as a first choice treatment. The drug is obviously effective but often too sedating, as indicated by its wide use as both an antidepressant and a sedative hypnotic. However, we have found that many patients cannot tolerate amitriptyline's marked anticholinergic side effects, which include a sense of spaciness that can occur more commonly with this drug, as well as marked dry mouth, constipation, etc.

With any of these drugs the clinician is best advised to start with a relatively low dose, which can then be increased slowly. For imipramine the starting doses and regimens vary. One common regimen is to prescribe 75 mg/day during week one, increasing weekly, as needed, to 150 mg/day during week two, 225 mg/day during week three, and 300 mg/day during week four. Another approach is to start at 50 mg/day, increasing the dose, as tolerated, by 25 mg/day to 150 mg/day and after some two weeks increasing from 150 mg at a rate of 50 mg every three days to 300 mg/day. (Similar dosage regimens are recommended for other uses of the drug—panic, pain, etc.) For some patients, particularly the elderly, it seems reasonable to begin at 25 mg on day one and increase to 50 mg on day two, allowing the patient to become acclimated to a single small dose. We also advise a more conservative schedule, remaining at 50 mg/day for one week and thereafter increasing the dosage at a rate of 25 mg every two days to 150 mg/day. After seven days on 150 mg/day, the dosage can be increased further as tolerated. The elderly present a somewhat unique problem (see Chapter 12). The not uncommon medical problems of the elderly and their relatively slow drug metabolism usually dictate conservative management; however, clinicians must be careful since some elderly patients are not slow metabolizers but instead require reasonably high dosages and run the risk of being undertreated. The degree of side effects can be a useful barometer as to the ability to tolerate a given dosage, and plasma levels may aid in prescribing optimal doses (see the sections below on Tricyclic Blood Levels and Side Effects).

For doxepin, amitriptyline, and trimipramine, dosage ranges similar to those for imipramine are recommended both in younger and older patients. We have recently been impressed with trimipramine's relatively low side effect profile in the elderly and with its rapid effects on promoting sleep. Nortriptyline and protriptyline are prescribed in rather different ways. In younger patients, protriptyline is generally started at 15 mg (5 mg TID) in week one with increases of 5-10 mg/week to a maximum of 60 mg/day. (In the elderly begin at 10 mg/day.) Nortriptyline, which is the only TCA to clearly have a so-called therapeutic window, can be ineffective if the patient attains either too low or too high plasma levels. The therapeutic dosage range for nortriptyline in adults is 50-150 mg/day. We recommend starting at 50 mg/day and increasing at a rate of 50 mg/week. (In the elderly begin at 25 mg/day and increase to 50 mg/day after three or four days.) After three weeks, a decrease in dosage may actually be helpful, a state of affairs rather different from the other

TCAs (see the section on Tricyclic Blood Levels). Amoxapine's starting dose in healthy adults is 150 mg/day with a maximum daily dose of 400 mg/day. Maprotiline's starting and maximum dosages are 75 and 225 mg/day, respectively. To avoid seizures, the starting dose of maprotiline should be maintained for two weeks and after six weeks of treatment, the dosage should be reduced to a maximum of 175 mg/day.

The response to TCAs is slower than one would hope. Traditionally, the rule of thumb has been that it takes two weeks for patients to begin to respond and that patients who are going to respond will begin to show some positive effects by four weeks. (One notable exception is amoxapine, which may work in as little as four days and enjoys a claim for more rapid onset.) Quitkin et al. (1984) reviewed a large series of depressed patients who were treated with traditional tricyclic antidepressants and concluded that relatively few patients demonstrate significant improvement after only two weeks of therapy and many require as long as six weeks to respond. Our group has reported that slow and rapid responders to maprotiline could be identified biologically by their pretreatment urinary levels of 3-methoxy-4-hydroxy-phenylglycol (MHPG), which is indicative of norepinephrine function. Patients with low MHPG levels demonstrate rapid responses (in less than 14 days), and those with very high MHPG levels need four to six weeks of treatment.

What should the clinician do if after six weeks the patient has either demonstrated a partial response or has not responded at all? First, the clinician should consider increasing dosage (except if the maximum maprotiline dose has been attained), since some patients are rapid—and not slow—drug metabolizers. Here, too, plasma levels can be a guide for increasing the dosage and determining how high to go (see section on Tricyclic Blood Levels). For other patients, the addition of lithium carbonate or Cytomel (T_3) can bring out a clinical response (see the section on Combination Therapies). If these additions do not produce a response, the clinician is faced with the option of either changing the drug or moving on to electroconvulsive therapy. For many years and still today in many centers, clinicians will choose to switch from one TCA to another. Increasingly, we have become dissatisfied with this approach. Our experience has been that patients who have tolerated, but have not responded to, an adequate trial on one tricyclic will rarely respond to an adequate trial of a second. All too often we have seen patients who have had multiple unsuccessful TCA trials. We recommend switching to another class of treatment sooner than was previously common.

If the patient responds, how long should he or she stay on the drug? Here, too, clinical thinking has changed. Early practice was to keep patients on the drug for a few months. Currently, practice has moved to longer term maintenance treatment of at least six to 12 months to prevent early relapse. In a recent major NIMH collaborative study (Prien et al. 1984), imipramine was generally more effective than placebo or lithium in preventing relapse of major depression over a two-year maintenance. In contrast to this study, two earlier major studies, here and in the United Kingdom, found lithium to be as effective as the tricyclic in preventing relapses in unipolar depressed patients. In the study by Prien et al. (1984), the overall relapse rate in the unipolar group was relatively high (overall relapse rate = 64 percent; imipramine group = 49 percent), and the authors even argued for the need to develop newer, alternative strategies, perhaps with drugs other than tricyclic antidepressants. (For further discussion of maintenance therapy in affective disorders, see Chapter 4).

After being maintained for some three to four months on the doses at which they responded, many patients can be maintained at lower doses (one-half to three-quarters that of the original dose) for the remaining months. If symptoms reemerge, dosage should be restored to the previous level if possible. If the patient begins to relapse on the same dose to which he or she had previously responded, the addition of 25 μg/day of Cytomel will often bring about a renewed response (see Chapter 9). Another option is to recheck the plasma level: if it isn't high, the dosage can be increased to bring the plasma level into the so-called therapeutic range (see below). This area is a confusing one for the clinician and patient, who naturally wonder whether the drug's effect has worn off or a natural recurrence has taken place.

Fortunately, maintenance on tricyclics or other antidepressants is generally not associated with particular major long-term side effects in contrast to those seen with lithium (thyroid goiter) or antipsychotics (tardive dyskinesia). (Again, maprotiline's maintenance dosage should not exceed 200 mg/day.) However, as described below, long-term use of the MAOIs does pose a cumulative, increased risk for acute hypertensive crises occurring (see below) should a patient unsuspectedly ingest certain foodstuffs or other medications. Also, alprazolam used for prolonged periods can possibly result in dependence (see Chapter 6).

When discontinuing or tapering tricyclics, it is most prudent to do so at a rate of 25 mg every two to three days. Many patients will demonstrate symptoms of cholinergic rebound if the TCA is discontinued too abruptly. These include nausea, queasy stomach, sweating, headache, neck pain, vomiting, etc. Moreover, we reported that some patients will demonstrate "rebound" hypomania or mania with sudden cessation of TCAs, an observation confirmed by others.

When the issue of rebound symptoms versus a medical illness or recurrence of psychiatric symptoms is in doubt, a single dose of the discontinued drug will often relieve the symptoms rapidly, confirming the diagnosis of a withdrawal syndrome. There is one report in which withdrawal mania responded to reinstitution of desipramine therapy.

Tricyclic Blood Levels

In recent years, increasing attention has been paid to the use of drug blood levels to monitor treatment with various psychotropic agents. Currently blood levels are most commonly used in patients treated with tricyclic antidepressants, neuroleptics, lithium carbonate, and anticonvulsants. Blood levels for benzodiazepines are neither widely available nor commonly used. Drug concentrations are determined primarily in serum (lithium carbonate, anticonvulsants) or plasma (tricyclic antidepressants). In addition to measuring the concentration of neuroleptics in blood, some laboratories also measure the relative binding to dopamine receptors (so-called radioreceptor assays).

Generally, blood levels are determined in blood drawn eight to 12 hours after the patient's last dose in an effort to avoid "false" peaks in blood levels that would occur if blood was drawn immediately after a patient has taken the medication. Also, plasma levels are most accurate when drawn after the patient has achieved "steady state"—the point at which a specific dose of drug given over a several-day period produces a consistent blood level. For TCAs this is approximately five to seven days.

Plasma levels can be particularly useful barometers of drug metabolism. There is approximately a 30-fold difference among human subjects in plasma levels of tricyclic antidepressants produced by a single fixed mg/kg dose of a drug, reflecting the degree to which the slowest and fastest metabolizers differ in drug absorption and metabolism. Obviously, slow metabolizers (such as the elderly) are at a higher risk for becoming toxic; fast metabolizers may have difficulty building drug levels. Most patients, however, fall in the middle range of the normal bell-shaped curve distribution.

For tricyclic antidepressants, the clearest use is in patients with endogenous depression. There is little or no relationship between TCA level and clinical response in patients with nonendogenous depression or those with dysthymia. Two types of relationships between TCA levels and clinical response in endogenously depressed patients have been described in the literature. Glassman et al. (1977) have reported a sigmoidal relationship between response and imipramine

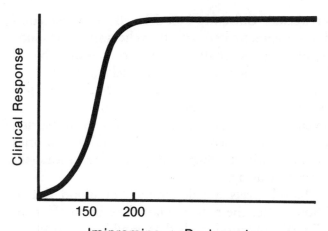

Figure 3-2. Sigmoidal Relationship Between Clinical Response and Imipramine Plus Desipramine Plasma Levels

plus desipramine levels; clinical response increases with plasma level up to ~250 ng/ml and then levels off thereafter (Figure 3-2). Glassman has reported rates of response of 30 percent, 67 percent, and 93 percent for patients with plasma levels in the following ranges: <150, 150-225, and >225 ng/ml. For nortriptyline, a curvilinear relationship has been described as indicated in Figure 3-3. Response increases with plasma level and then plateaus in a range of ~50-150 ng/ml with a decrease in response at plasma levels >150 ng/ml. The critical 50-150 ng/ml range has been called the therapeutic window. Nonresponding patients with plasma levels of ~150 ng/ml may respond to a lowering of dosage and plasma level into the window. The decreased responsivity above the window is not due to side effects. Therapeutic windows have at times been described for other drugs, but these are not as clear as with nortriptyline. Approximate therapeutic plasma levels are summarized in Table 3-D.

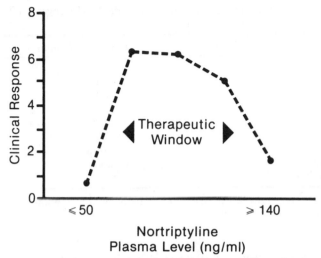

Figure 3-3. Curvilinear Relationship Between Clinical Response and Nortriptyline Plasma Levels

A number of medications may increase or decrease plasma levels—generally by interfering with or augmenting liver microsomal enzyme activity. For example, nicotine, barbiturates (including Fiorinal), chloral hydrate, phenytoin, and carbamazepine induce breakdown of TCAs, and clinicians should keep this in mind when prescribing TCAs to patients who are taking the above compounds. In contrast, antipsychotics (particularly phenothiazines), methylphenidate, disulfiram, and fenfluramine will increase plasma levels by slowing drug metabolism in the liver.

Conversely, tricyclics increase phenothiazine plasma levels as well. Benzodiazepines and antiparkinsonian medications have little or no effect on TCA levels.

A number of issues arise when one considers plasma level data. For one, studies generally use fixed mg/kg dosaging such that it is possible that a patient with a given TCA plasma level (e.g., 250 ng/ml) on a given dose (e.g., 300 mg/

Table 3-D. Approximate Therapeutic Plasma Level Ranges for Tricyclic and Tetracyclic Drugs

Drug	Blood Level (ng/ml)
amitriptyline	100–250*
desipramine	150–300
doxepin	120–250*
imipramine	150–300*
nortriptyline†	50–150
protriptyline	75–250
trimipramine	Unknown
amoxapine	Unknown
maprotiline	150–250

* Total concentration of drug and demethylated metabolite.
† Has a clear therapeutic window.

day of imipramine) might well have responded to a lower dosage and at a lower plasma level. In a sense, then, plasma levels can be viewed as barometers of adequacy of treatment. Patients who are not responding to a four- to six-week trial of imipramine but who have attained a plasma level of 150 ng/ml or less may respond to an increase in dosage and plasma level to >200 ng/ml. On the other hand, another patient who is responding at exactly the same dosage and plasma level does not need to have the dosage or plasma level increased even if it is below the therapeutic range. Some investigators have advocated determining the plasma level for any patient who is responding to a tricyclic so as to record *that patient's* therapeutic plasma level on that drug. This could prove important if the patient has a later recurrence and requires retreatment.

Sometimes a routine check of a tricyclic blood level in a patient who is clinically much improved and has only minor side effects will reveal a plasma level of >400 ng/ml, and the patient will relapse when the dose is decreased to bring down the plasma level. This result suggests that, for that particular patient, a very high plasma level was necessary for improvement.

So far, only amitriptyline shows clear toxicity related to

plasma levels around 500 ng/ml. Obviously, clinical judgment is necessary. The EKG may be useful in patients who do well only on very high plasma levels to make sure cardiac conduction is not seriously affected.

Another practical problem has revolved around the variation among laboratories in their tricyclic assays. This is of major importance since clinicians may be unable to interpret a given value in their laboratories. A major national effort is underway to cross-validate laboratories, and eventually this problem should be resolved. Physicians should check with their laboratories as to whether quality control methods are being routinely employed. At any rate, plasma levels can provide useful clinical information if the clinician keeps these issues in mind.

Side Effects

A review of *PDR* package insert information on each of the TCAs and related agents points to their exerting a myriad of side effects. These can be grouped broadly by categories: e.g., anticholinergic, autonomic, allergic, etc. (Table 3-C). This organization is somewhat artificial, since a single side effect (e.g., sedation) may actually be due to any number of distinct neurochemical effects (e.g., histamine blockade, increased serotonin availability, and others, or combinations thereof). In addition, some side effects may reflect drug action either in the brain or in the periphery or in both (e.g., orthostatic hypotension).

How can clinicians help in the management of side effects? In some patients, particularly those with complicating medical illnesses, side reactions may not be entirely controllable or manageable. There are, however, some things that can be done, particularly for less severe reactions in medically healthy patients.

One very important issue is attitude. Not uncommonly, some psychiatrists have rather negative views about medication, and these can be communicated indirectly or overtly, particularly if the impetus to try medications has arisen from the patient and not the physician. In our experience, this attitude can be troubling to the patient, who must rely on the physician's belief in the importance of medication trials and in being able to deal with the side effects. It is thus imperative for clinicians to develop well-reasoned and balanced views about drug prescribing.

A general principle of drug prescribing is that some side effects can be managed by reducing dosage or can be avoided by increasing it slowly. In our experience this is particularly true for the early emergence of "spaciness," depersonalization, confusion, orthostatic hypotension, or marked sedation. If these reactions persist in the presence of more moderate dose escalation, a switch to another TCA may be necessary. In dealing with anticholinergic side effects or sedation, switching to desipramine seems reasonable. For patients who develop orthostatic hypotension, nortriptyline is often a useful alternative, since it tends to produce orthostatic changes at plasma levels above the so-called therapeutic window. Thus it is more easily tolerated than imipramine whose orthostatic effects are often produced at low plasma levels (see the preceding section on Tricyclic Blood Levels).

Peripheral anticholinergic side effects have also been reported to be ameliorated by administering bethanechol, a procholinergic drug, in doses of 25 to 50 mg given three or four times daily. Generally this is continued for as long as the patient remains on tricyclic antidepressant. This drug can be particularly helpful to patients with urinary hesitancy. For dry mouth, various dental mouthwash preparations that contain the cholinergic agent pilocarpine can be quite helpful. These mouthwashes are not widely available but can be obtained from some pharmacists, psychopharmacologists or dentists. In cases of anticholinergic deliria, physostigmine (a centrally acting procholinergic agent) may be administered either iv or im to clarify the diagnosis. (For specific information regarding the use of physostigmine, see Chapter 9.)

An important antihistaminic effect is weight gain—particularly seen with amitriptyline and doxepin—which can be difficult to control pharmacologically. Often, patients who demonstrate this side effect on one TCA will continue to gain weight when switched to another related drug. In some patients, switching to trazodone, bupropion, or—when available—to fluoxetine may be the only way to maintain an antidepressant effect and promote weight reduction (see sections below), since MAOIs will also cause weight gain. Unfortunately, there are patients who still continue to gain weight while receiving the drug to which they are showing an antidepressant response. In such cases, support and advice regarding dieting may be the only recourse.

Two of the newer compounds—maprotiline and amoxapine—have been reported to produce troublesome side effects—seizures and extrapyramidal symptoms—that have been less frequently reported with the standard TCAs. Induced seizures have been reported in a number of single case reports using maprotiline. Recently, our group reported a series of 11 seizure patients at one hospital as well as a study of all U.S. maprotiline-related seizures. In our series, prolonged treatment (greater than six weeks) at high dosages (200 to 400 mg/day) appeared to be a major factor. This was confirmed in the U.S. survey. In addition, rapid dose escalation—reaching 150 mg/day within seven days—was a major factor in the general survey. When these two factors were eliminated, the risk of seizures appeared to approximate that associated with classic antidepressants (~0.2 percent). The manufacturer has altered its dosage guidelines, recommending beginning at 75 mg/day for two weeks, a maximum dose of 225 mg/day for up to six weeks, and maintenance at 200 mg/day or below. The previous dosage schedule had been similar to that of imipramine.

Amoxapine has been reported to produce a number of side effects associated with dopamine receptor blockade—e.g., galactorrhea, akathisia, and other extrapyramidal symptoms—and even a few cases of dyskinesia, similar to those more commonly found with the neuroleptic loxapine. Amoxapine is metabolized generally to a 7-OH metabolite. In some individuals, alternate hydroxylation at the 8 position results in the accumulation of a neuroleptic metabolite. Generally speaking, we recommend tapering or stopping medications if these symptoms occur (see the preceding section on Tricyclic Blood Levels).

MONOAMINE OXIDASE INHIBITORS (MAOIS)

The primary *PDR* clinical indication for monoamine oxidase inhibitors (MAOIs) is for depression that is refractory to tricyclic therapy. Phenelzine enjoys an indication for anxious depression. Although the British have emphasized frequently that the MAOIs are not particularly helpful in endogenous depression, the American experience, including our own, has been entirely different. These drugs have been life savers for many endogenously depressed patients, particularly those who have failed to respond to TCAs.

Why the discrepancy? For one, there is little doubt that MAOIs are effective in patients with panic attacks or with anxious or atypical depression. However, their effectiveness in endogenous depression may require the prescription of considerably higher dosages than the early British trials, which used relatively low dosages. Another difficulty with determining ranges of efficacy revolves around the occurrence of pronounced obsessionality, agitation, and anxiety in many endogenously depressed patients who may be misdiagnosed as atypically depressed. Interestingly, several investigators have reported an association between severity, anxiety, and platelet MAO activity in endogenously depressed patients, suggesting that high MAO levels might prove to be a marker

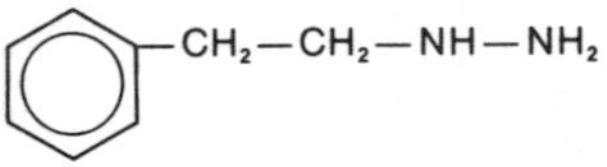

Phenelzine 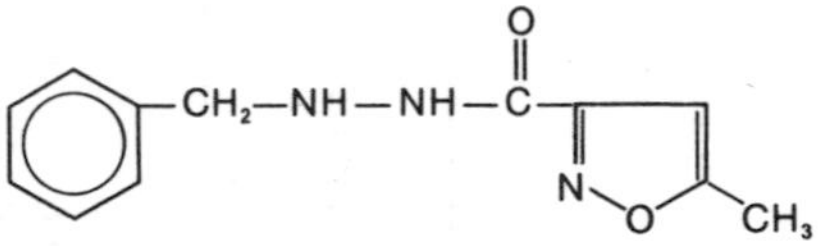   Isocarboxazid

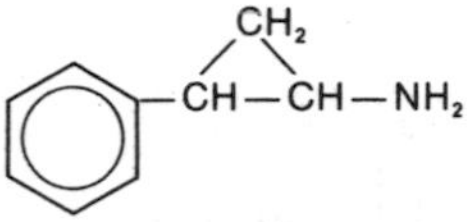

Tranylcypromine

Figure 3-4. Chemical Structures of Monoamine Oxidase
Inhibitors

for deciding which patients will respond to MAOIs and for
clarifying the delineation between endogenous and nonendogenous depression.

There are two structural classes of MAOIs: the hydra-
zines—isocarboxazid and phenelzine—and the nonhydra-
zine—tranylcypromine (see Figure 3-4 and Table 3-E).

Dosages

The dosages of the three drugs are dissimilar. The traditional therapeutic ranges follow: isocarboxazid, 20 to 30 mg/
day; phenelzine, 45 to 90 mg/day; and tranylcypromine, 30
to 50 mg/day. Most patients will require treatment at the
higher dosages. For example, 90 mg/day of phenelzine is
commonly required in a patient with severe depressive illness.

A patient treated with phenelzine should be started at 30
mg/day and increased to 45 mg/day after three days. Thereafter, dosage can be increased at a rate of 15 mg/week to 90
mg/day. We have seen patients who require as much as 120
mg/day; however, many patients cannot tolerate the orthostatic side effects of these drugs. Some investigators have

Table 3-E. Monoamine Oxidase Inhibitors (MAOIs) and Other Available Drugs

Generic Name	Brand Name	Tablets	Oral Concentrate	Parenteral	Usual Therapeutic Dosages (mg/day)*
MAOIs					
isocarboxazid	Marplan	10 mg	None	None	30–50
phenelzine	Nardil	15 mg	None	None	45–90
tranylcypromine	Parnate	10 mg	None	None	30–50
Other					
trazodone	Desyrel	50/100 mg	None	None	150–300
buproprion	Wellbutrin	75/100 mg	None	None	200–450

*These dosage ranges are approximate. Many patients will respond at relatively low dosages (even below ranges given above); others may require higher dosages.

Table 3-F. Common or Troublesome Side Effects of Monoamine Oxidase Inhibitors

1. Orthostatic hypotension
2. Hypertensive crises (interactions with foodstuffs or medications)
3. Hyperpyrexic reactions
4. Anorgasmia or sexual impotence
5. Sedation (particularly daytime and due to no. 6)
6. Insomnia during night
7. Stimulation during day
8. Muscle cramps and myositic-like reactions
9. Urinary hesitancy
10. Constipation
11. Dry mouth
12. Weight gain
13. Myoclonic twitches

recommended 1 mg/kg per day dose of the drug as a guideline for adequacy of treatment.

For tranylcypromine, a starting dose of 20 mg/day for three days seems reasonable. This can then be increased to 30 mg/day for one week with 10 mg/day increases to 50 to 60 mg/day. The current recommended maximum dose of the drug is 40 mg/day. Isocarboxazid, which is less commonly prescribed than the others, should be titrated at a rate similar to that for tranylcypromine. Its recommended maximum daily dosage is 30 mg/day, and the manufacturer indicates it can be started at that dose as well. Higher doses, up to 50 mg/day, have been required for some patients. Once a patient has responded, the medication should be maintained for a similar length of time comparable to that recommended for the tricyclics.

Side Effects

Common side effects are listed in Table 3-F. Since MAOIs are not purported to block acetylcholine receptors, they produce less in the way of dry mouth, blurred vision, constipation, and urinary hesitancy. However, we have seen patients who have developed urinary hesitancy, presumably on the basis of an increase in noradrenergic activity. When it occurs, a reduction in dosage may help. We have been less impressed with the adjunctive use of bethanecol with MAOIs than with TCAs.

The most common side effect is dizziness, particularly of the orthostatic type. This appears to be somewhat more common with MAOIs than with TCAs. Dose reduction may help, but again we have often found this to be a problem, since too great a reduction in dose may lead to reemergence of depressive symptoms. Several approaches include a) maintenance of adequate hydration—about eight glasses of fluid a day—and increased salt intake; b) support stockings, bellybinders, or corsets; and c) addition of a mineralocorticoid (Florinef). Although this mineralocorticoid has been used in patients with orthostatic hypotension not induced by medication, we have rarely found it helpful in usual daily doses of 0.3 mg. We have been told by colleagues that Florinef can be effective at total daily doses of 0.6-0.8 mg. An intriguing report recently appeared pointing to the use of small amounts of cheese to help maintain blood pressure—a counterintuitive but imaginative solution. However, most clinicians are likely to be wary of the understandable risk of hypertensive crises with cheese, particularly when one does not really know the tyramine content of the foodstuff. Similarly, one would intuit that adding a stimulant (dextroamphetamine or methylphenidate) to an MAOI would result in marked surges of blood pressure. In fact, however, Feighner et al. (1985) reported that the addition of stimulants for patients receiving MAOIs or MAOI/TCA combinations normalized blood pressure in depressed patients with serious orthostatic hypotension, or brought out a clinical response in previously nonresponsive patients. There were no incidences of hypertensive crises; in fact, several of the patients developed orthostatic hypotension. Daily dosages used were 5-20 mg of *d*-amphetamine and 10-15 mg of methylphenidate. They recommend beginning at

2.5 mg/day of either drug. We have also heard of several clinicians in the community who have used these approaches successfully.

The greatest side-effect problems involve untoward interactions with certain foodstuffs or cold remedies, which may produce hypertensive crises with violent headaches and occasional cerebrovascular accidents, or hyperpyrexic states that can lead to coma. MAO in the intestinal tract degrades tyramine. When inhibited by MAOIs, the individual is at risk for absorbing large amounts of tyramine, which can act as a false neurotransmitter or an indirect agonist and elevate blood pressure. Fortunately, dietary restrictions can markedly reduce the risk. Various prohibited foods are included in lists in *PDR*. These lists have been reviewed by several investigators, and relative risks have been attributed to many of them (Table 3-G).

Of particular importance regarding medication interactions is warning the patient *not* to take other medications along with the MAOIs unless first checking with the physician. Demerol, epinephrine, local anesthetics (containing antihistamines) and decongestants can be particularly dangerous.

If a patient develops a surge in blood pressure with violent headaches, he or she should be instructed to go to a local emergency room. Phentolamine (Regitine), a central alpha blocker, can be administered intravenously to reverse the acute rise in blood pressure. Some psychopharmacologists have recommended that patients take oral chlorpromazine when headache occurs. We have tended not to do this if patients have not had a documented increase in blood pressure, because some patients will display marked headaches secondary to a lowering of blood pressure. We advise patients with headaches to have their blood pressure checked. Also, routine monitoring of blood pressure, particularly during the first six weeks, seems prudent (for both the drug's hypotensive and hypertensive effects).

Sedation and activation are also potential problems, the

Table 3-G.   Foods to Be Avoided with Monoamine Oxidase Inhibitors*

Foods definitely to be avoided:
  Beer, red wine
  Aged cheeses (cottage and cream cheese are allowed)
  Dry sausage
  Fava or Italian green beans
  Brewer's yeast
  Smoked fish
  Liver (beef or chicken)

Foods that may cause problems in large amounts but are otherwise less problematic:
  Alcohol
  Ripe avocado
  Sour cream
  Yogurt
  Bananas (ripe)
  ? Soy sauce

Foods that were thought to be problems but are probably not problematic in usual quantities:
  Chocolate
  Figs
  Meat tenderizers
  Caffeine-containing beverages
  Raisins

* Based on McCabe B, Tsuang MT: Dietary considerations in MAO inhibitor regimens. *J Clin Psychiatry* 43:178–181, 1982.

latter being more common. Activation takes two forms: stimulation during the day (particularly with tranylcypromine) and insomnia at night. Tranylcypromine's stimulatory effects have been related to its having a structure similar to that of amphetamines, although this pharmacologic link has not been clearly established. Overstimulation can be ameliorated somewhat by dose reduction, although the side effect is not easily eliminated. If a dose reduction does not result in a decrease in stimulation, patients may require being switched to another medication.

Phenelzine overall is far less stimulating and more sedative than is tranylcypromine. As such it offers a major alternative for daytime overstimulation. However, phenelzine may produce both insomnia and secondary daytime sedation. Oddly, one often encounters insomnia in patients who are nevertheless showing a good clinical response, making it a particularly difficult side effect to manage. Changing the dosage regimen may be helpful. Patients who are not taking phenelzine in the evening may benefit from switching the drug to evening hours. Conversely, patients who are taking much of the drug in the evening may respond by moving it to earlier in the day. These manipulations can be helpful, although in our experience they are highly variable in their efficacy. Some patients may ultimately require potent hypnotics to overcome persistent insomnia.

As the dose of an MAOI is increased to high levels in an attempt to achieve a therapeutic effect, patients occasionally become "intoxicated"—drunk, ataxic, confused, and sometimes euphoric. This is a sign of overdosage, and the dose should be reduced.

Some patients develop muscle pains or paresthesiae which are probably the result of the MAOI interfering with pyridoxine (vitamin B-6) metabolism. Pyridoxine administered in doses of approximately 100 mg/day can be helpful.

A particularly bothersome side effect is anorgasmia, which in some patients lessens over time. We have not been impressed with any pharmacologic attempts to counteract this side effect, although cyproheptadine (Periactin) has recently been said to be helpful.

If the clinician wishes to switch a patient from one MAOI to another, care must be taken to avoid drug-drug interactions. The clinician should taper the patient off one MAOI and allow for a 10- to 14-day drug-free period before beginning another MAOI. Some patients have experienced severe untoward reactions in switching from one MAOI to another, particularly from phenelzine to tranylcypromine, perhaps reflecting the latter's amphetamine-like properties.

When making a transition between tricyclic antidepressants and MAOIs, *PDR* recommends that patients be off all medications between trials for 10 to 14 days. Some clinicians, however, have reported that a briefer drug-free period of one to five days is sufficient when going from a TCA to an MAOI. When conversely going from an MAOI to a TCA, the 10- to 14-day period is generally recommended. The difference in these strategies is probably due to the 10- to 14-day period needed to regenerate MAO. Thus, even after stopping MAOIs, patients should be warned to follow their dietary restrictions for an additional 14 days.

Augmenting Response

L-Tryptophan (2 to 6 g/day) added to MAOIs has been shown to improve or speed clinical response in a few studies. L-Tryptophan might also help as a mild hypnotic. However, we have not found that adding this amino acid is particularly helpful, and rare adverse effects—such as tremor and confusion—have occurred in patients who are suddenly given 3 to 6 g of L-tryptophan on top of established MAO therapy.

If a patient fails to respond to MAOIs, a trial of lithium may be added to bring out a clinical response. Unlike the case of tricyclics, we have not found the addition of T_3 (Cytomel) helpful in augmenting clinical responsivity to MAOIs.

TRAZODONE

Trazodone is a new breed in the United States of an antidepressant introduced in Italy over a decade ago (Table 3-E). Its structure bears no resemblance to any of the other marketed antidepressants (Figure 3-5). However, it has a triazolo ring as does alprazolam (see Figure 6-1 in Chapter 6). It is a central serotonin reuptake blocker as well as having alpha norepinephrine receptor-blocking effects. Its pharmacology is complex, and its specific mode of action has not

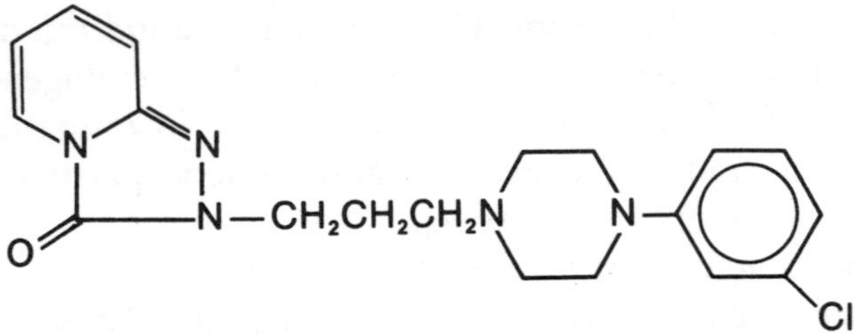

Trazodone

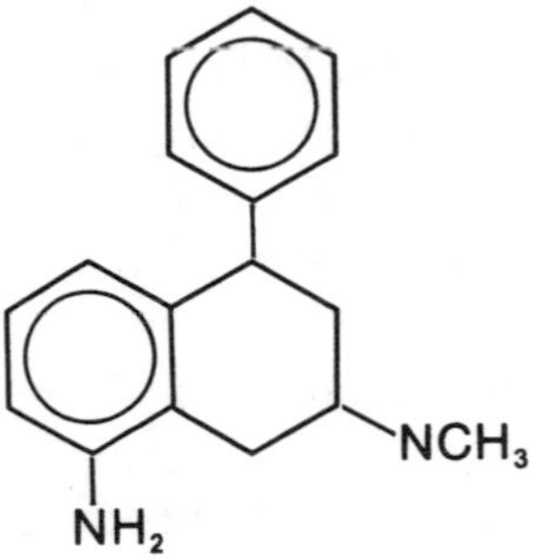

Nomifensine

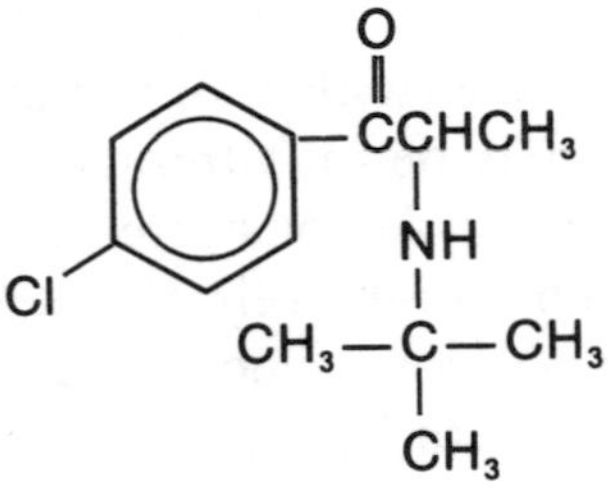

Bupropion

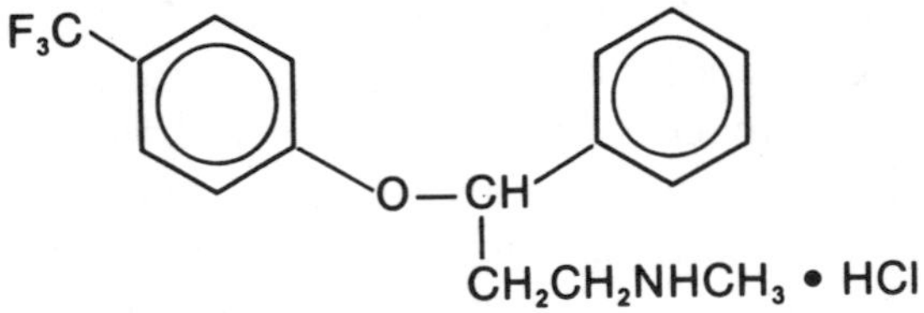

Fluoxetine

Figure 3-5. Chemical Structures of Other Antidepressants

been clearly described. Some clinicians have found the drug to be less potent than tricyclics and MAOIs in endogenous depression. We have found it most effective in outpatients with mild to moderate depression and anxiety, particularly those with difficulty falling asleep.

The manufacturer recommends starting patients at 150 mg/day and then increasing up to 600 mg/day (Table 3-E). Our experience has been that the drug is quite sedating, and we begin patients at 50 to 100 mg/day and increase to 150 mg/day by days three to five. Thereafter, we increase by 50 to 75 mg weekly to 300 mg/day. In our hands, patients respond at a modal dose of 150 to 300 mg/day. Indeed, some clinicians have proposed that trazodone has a therapeutic window: as with nortriptyline, too high plasma levels are associated with poor responses. Our experience would suggest this may be so, although the blood level studies done to date have not demonstrated any clear, rational relationships between blood levels and response.

Trazodone is not anticholinergic. It can, however, produce dry mouth because of its norepinephrine activity (salivation is controlled by both acetylcholine and norepinephrine systems). In addition to sedation, two side effects can be particularly troublesome. First, when taken on an empty stomach (particularly in high dosages), trazodone can produce acute dizziness and fainting. Patients should be warned to take the drug only after they have eaten. Some patients will also describe headaches or nausea rather than faintness if they take the drug on an empty stomach. Another reaction is priapism, with some 20 plus cases having been reported in the United States. This is rare but very problematic, with some patients requiring surgical intervention. If not treated successfully, priapism might result in impotence. This consequence is said to be averted if the priapism is treated within the first few hours. Male patients should thus be warned to stop the drug immediately if they experience any symptoms suggestive of priapism and to seek emergency room treatment if the erection persists longer than one hour.

Maintenance treatment with trazodone has been well studied in two trials. Patients have been reported to tolerate the drug well for prolonged periods. Generally, we have maintained patients at 75 to 100 percent of the dose to which they had responded, but clinicians may wish to try maintenance at 50 percent if side effects are noted.

ALPRAZOLAM

The triazolobenzodiazepine alprazolam is "approved" in patients with anxiety or anxiety associated with depression (see Figure 6-1). However, the drug appears to have potent antipanic effects and only moderate antidepressant effects. Unlike diazepam or other typical benzodiazepines, alprazolam appears to affect noradrenergic systems (see Chapter 6) and to have reasonable effects comparable to imipramine and doxepin in mildly to moderately depressed outpatients at doses from 1.5 mg/day to as high as 6 to 10 mg/day. Generally, mildly to moderately depressed outpatients require 1.5-4.0 mg/day. We recommend starting at 1.0-1.5 mg/day, increasing dosage by 0.5 mg every three days to 4.0 mg. The drug can be sedating, particularly in the patient previously not exposed to benzodiazepines. When stopping the drug, tapering is essential. Tapering is often done by a 0.5 mg reduction every three days. If the dosage is pushed too high and maintained for longer periods, discontinuation will take some time. This is a potential drawback to the drug.

Alprazolam's effects in seriously depressed endogenous patients are neither easily predictable nor consistent. It does appear to be an effective antidepressant in some patients with endogenous depression. For example, in one study of depressed inpatients with shortened rapid eye movement (REM) latency, the drug was not as effective as amitriptyline but was effective in some patients. Because its effects in endogenous depression are so highly variable, its usefulness as a primary treatment in this group is limited. Mooney et al. (1985) reported that alprazolam enhances signal transduction by the receptor/N-protein/adenylate cyclase enzyme complex, and this effect may be related to drug response. But these tests are research tools and are not readily available. (For further discussion of alprazolam see Chapter 6.)

NOMIFENSINE

Nomifensine is a multicyclic compound (Figure 3-5) with both dopamine and norepinephrine reuptake blocking effects, conferring upon it both antidepressant and mild stimulant-like properties. It had been available in West Germany for many years, and European colleagues advocated it for the more anergic patient. We have seen several such patients who had failed to respond to TCAs but who responded very well to this compound. Its usual dosage range was 100 to 200 mg/day. The starting dose was 100 mg/day with 50 mg/day increases to 200 to 300 mg/day (Table 3-E). Despite its short half-life (about two hours), studies indicated it could be given on a once-a-day basis, although twice a day (early morning and afternoon) was quite common. Since the drug may be stimulating, patients were advised not to take the drug beyond the late afternoon. Additional side effects included agitation, sedation (in some patients), headaches, and insomnia. The drug appeared to have a reasonable safety margin in cases of overdosage, making it less problematic in suicidal patients. In addition, it did not appear to lower seizure thresholds. In a relatively small percentage of patients (as high as 3-10 percent), the drug produced an allergic reaction characterized by flulike symptoms and fever, not uncommonly seen with other quinoline compounds. Generally, this syndrome abated with discontinuation of the drug. It also produced mild elevations in blood pressure, particularly in patients on other sympathomimetic agents, as well as hemolytic anemia and elevations in liver enzymatic activity. The manufacturer recommended periodic blood counts and liver-function tests in patients treated with the drug. However, because in Great Britian there had been a small number of deaths secondary to hemolytic anemias, the manufacturer discontinued the drug in early 1986. Conceivably, it could reappear on the U.S market in the future.

BUPROPION

Bupropion is a unicyclic (Figure 3-5) that is about to be released. This drug is not a norepinephrine drug or serotonin reuptake blocker, nor does it inhibit monoamine oxidase. Its biochemical mode of action is unclear, although it has been hypothesized to act via dopamine reuptake blockade. This remains moot since its dopamine potentiating effects in animals appear to occur at very high dosages and blood levels, well beyond those expected in humans. Moreover, when dopamine effects were demonstrated in humans in one study, they appeared to be related to possible psychotic reactions on the drug rather than to its antidepressant responses. The drug appears effective in patients with depression but not in those with panic-related disorders.

Bupropion has a relatively wide usual dosage range of 150 to 450 mg/day (see Table 3-E). The modal optimum dosage range in our hands has been 300-400 mg/day. It has a favorable side-effect profile since it is not anticholinergic. Its side effects have appeared to us to be nonspecific in the patients we have treated over the past few years, although nausea occurs in occasional patients, and rare seizures have been reported by others. It does not induce orthostatic hypotension or stimulate appetite. Some have argued that the drug could be particularly useful in patients who gain weight while receiving TCAs. However, recent experience with newly marketed drugs has pointed out that only wide clinical use can be the ultimate test of how to use the drugs and what their limitations and side effects will be.

FLUOXETINE

Fluoxetine (Prozac) is one of a new group of antidepressant drugs that selectively inhibit the reuptake of serotonin. Its chemical structure is depicted in Figure 3-5. The drug was not approved by the FDA at the time of publication of this manual, but it has been extensively studied under double-blind conditions. Other specific serotonin reuptake blockers are in active clinical trials (e.g., Sertraline) but are not reportedly close to the U.S. market.

Fluoxetine exerts little effect on norepinephrine or dopamine reuptake in rat brain synaptosomes. In contrast, it is a potent serotonin reuptake blocker; its serotonin reuptake blocking effects are approximately 100 times those on norepinephrine or dopamine reuptake. The drug is 15 to 60 times a more potent serotonin reuptake blocker than is amitriptyline or doxepin. In contrast to fluoxetine's selective serotonin effects, amitriptyline and doxepin in similar models are equipotent in their norepinephrine and serotonin activity. Fluoxetine potently antagonizes brain serotonin—but not cardiac norepinephrine—depletion in mice treated with p-chloramphetamine and 6-OH dopamine, respectively. Interestingly, in this same model amitriptyline, doxepin, and trazodone did not reverse serotonin depletion, although they did exert serotonin reuptake blocking effects in the rat brain synaptosome model described above. Fluoxetine exerts very little effect on blocking muscarinic anticholinergic, histamine (H_1), serotonin ($5\text{-}HT_1$ and $5\text{-}HT_2$), and alpha$_1$ and alpha$_2$ norepinephrine receptors.

Fluoxetine's half-life is approximately one to three days; that of its demethylated metabolite, seven to 15 days. It does not alter the pharmacokinetic properties of anticonvulsants, chlorthiazide, or diazepam, nor does it increase blood concentrations of ethanol. Psychometric studies indicate that it does not enhance ethanol's effects on neurometric or psychomotor performance.

A number of double-blind studies have demonstrated it to be of equal efficacy to doxepin, amitriptyline, and desipramine, and to be significantly more effective than placebo, in the treatment of patients with major depression. The drug is initiated at 20 mg/day with increases to 40 mg/day for days two to four, 60 mg/day on days five to seven. The maximum recommended daily dosage of 80 mg/day can be attained by day eight. Many patients appear to respond well at dosages of 60 mg/day or less. The drug will be available in both 20 mg and 40 mg capsules.

Fluoxetine's side effect profile is generally more favorable than that of the tricyclic antidepressant drugs. It produces much less in the way of orthostatic hypotension, constipation, and dry mouth, appearing quite similar to placebo in the incidence of these side reactions. Its major side effects are nausea, tremor, drowsiness, sweating, headache, and nervousness. Unlike most tricyclics, it appears to facilitate weight loss and does not appear to potentiate seizures in humans. Last, it appears relatively safe in overdosages. One fatality was reported in the double-blind clinical trials in a patient who had also taken a number of other potentially lethal substances. There have been a few overdoses in the clinical trials on fluoxetine alone, but none of these reportedly resulted in fatalities. Thus, the drug appears to offer an advantage in this area over TCAs and MAOIs, although broader clinical use will ultimately be needed to fully map out its side effects profile and limits of safety.

Bibliography

Ambrusini PJ: A pharmacological paradigm for urinary incontinence and enuresis. J Clin Psychopharmacol 4:247–253, 1984

Asberg M, Cronholm B, Sjoqvist F, et al: Relationship between plasma level and therapeutic effect of nortriptyline. Br Med J 3:331–334, 1971

Bielski RJ, Friedel RO: Prediction of tricyclic antidepressant response: a critical review. Arch Gen Psychiatry 33:1479–1489, 1976

Blackwell B, Marley E, Price J, et al: Hypertensive interactions between monoamine oxidase inhibitors and foodstuffs. Br J Psychiatry 113:349, 1967

Cohen B, Harris P, Altesman R: Amoxapine: neuroleptic as well as an antidepressant? Am J Psychiatry 139:1165–1167, 1982

Cohn JP, Varga L, Lyford A: A two-center double-blind study of nomifensine, imipramine, and placebo in depressed geriatric outpatients. J Clin Psychiatry 45(4, sec 2):68–72, 1984

Cohn JP, Wilcox C: A comparison of fluoxetine, imipramine, and placebo in patients with major depressive disorder. J Clin Psychiatry 46(3, sec 2):26–31, 1985

Cole JO, Schatzberg AF, Sniffin C, et al: Trazodone in treatment-resistant depression: an open study. J Clin Psychopharm 1(Suppl 6):49–54, 1981

Cole JO, Schatzberg AF: Antidepressant drug therapy, in Psychiatry Update, vol 2. Edited by Grinspoon L. Washington, DC, American Psychiatric Press, 1983, pp 472–491, 542–544

Crane GE: Iproniazid (Marsilid) phosphate: a therapeutic agent for mental disorders and debilitating diseases. Psychiatry Research Reports 8:142–152, 1957

Dessain EC, Schatzberg AF, Woods BT, et al: Maprotiline treatment in depression: a perspective on seizures. Arch Gen Psychiatry (in press)

Feighner JP, Aden GC, Fabre LF, et al: Comparison of alprazolam, imipramine and placebo in the treatment of depression. JAMA 249:3056–3064, 1983

Feighner JP, Merideth CH, Claghorn JL: Multi-center placebo-controlled evaluation of nomifensine treatment in depressed outpatients. J Clin Psychiatry 45(4, sec 2):12–20, 1984

Feighner JP, Herbstein J, Damlouji N: Combined MAOI, TCA, and direct stimulant therapy of treatment-resistant depression. J Clin Psychiatry 46:206–209, 1985

Glassman A, Perel J: The clinical pharmacology of imipramine. Arch Gen Psychiatry 28:649–653, 1973

Glassman AH, Perel JM, Shostak M, et al: Clinical implications of imipramine plasma levels for depressive illness. Arch Gen Psychiatry 34:197–204, 1977

Kline NS: Clinical experience with iproniazid (Marsilid). Journal of Clinical and Experimental Psychopathology 19:72–78, 1958

Kuhn R: Uber die behandlung depressiver zustande mit einem iminodibenzylderivat (G22355). Schweiz Med Wochenschr 87:1135–1140, 1957

Lemberger L, Bergstrom RF, Wolen RL, et al: Fluoxetine: Clinical pharmacology and physiology disposition. J Clin Psychiatry 46(3, sec 2):14–19, 1985

Liebowitz MR, Quitkin FM, Stewart JW: Phenelzine v imipramine in atypical depression. Arch Gen Psychiatry 41:669–677, 1984

Mangla JC, Pereira M: Tricyclic antidepressants in the treatment of peptic ulcer disease. Arch Intern Med 142:273–275, 1982

McCabe B, Tsuang MT: Dietary consideration in MAO inhibitor regiments. J Clin Psychiatry 43:178–181, 1982

McGrath PJ, Quitkin FM, Harrison W, et al: Treatment of melancholia with tranylcypromine. Am J Psychiatry 141:288–289, 1984

Mirin SM, Schatzberg AF, Creasey DE: Hypomania and mania after tricyclic withdrawal. Am J Psychiatry 138:87–89, 1981

Mooney JJ, Schatzberg AF, Cole JO, et al: Enhanced signal transduction by adenylate cyclase in platelet membranes of patients showing antidepressant responses to alprazolam: preliminary data. J Psychiatr Res 19:65–75, 1985

Pope HG, Hudson JI, Jonas JM, et al: Bulimia treated with imipramine: a placebo-controlled, double-blind study. Am J Psychiatry 140:554–558, 1983

Preskorn S: Antidepressant response and plasma concentration of bupropion. J Clin Psychiatry 44(5, sec 2):137–139, 1983

Prien RF, Kupfer DJ, Mansky PA, et al: Drug therapy in the prevention of recurrences in unipolar and bipolar affective disorders. Arch Gen Psychiatry 41:1096–1104, 1984

Quitkin F, Rabkin A, Klein DF: Monoamine oxidase inhibitors. Arch Gen Psychiatry 36:749–760, 1979

Quitkin FM, Rabkin JG, Ross D, et al: Duration of antidepressant drug treatment: what is an adequate trial? Arch Gen Psychiatry 41:238–245, 1984

Rappoport JL, Mikkelsen EJ, Zavadil A, et al: Childhood enuresis, II: psychopathology, tricyclic concentration in plasma and antienuretic effect. Arch Gen Psychiatry 37:1146–1152, 1980

Ravaris CL, Nies A, Robinson DS, et al: A multiple-dose controlled study of phenelzine in depression-anxiety states. Arch Gen Psychiatry 33:347–350, 1976

Richelson E: The use of tricyclic antidepressants in chronic gastrointestinal pain. J Clin Psychiatry 43:50–55, 1982

Richelson E: Antimuscarinic and other receptor-blocking properties of antidepressants. Mayo Clin Proc 58:40–46, 1983

Rickels K, Smith WT, Blandin V, et al: Comparison of two dosage regimens of fluoxetine in major depression. J Clin Psychiatry 46(3, sec 2):38–41, 1985

Robinson DS, Nies A, Ravaris CL, et al: Clinical pharmacology of phenelzine. Arch Gen Psychiatry 35:629–635, 1978

Robinson DS, Kayser A, Corcella J, et al: Hyperphagia, hypersomnia, panic attacks, hysterical traits, and somatic anxiety predict phenelzine response in depressed outpatients. Presented at Annual Meeting of the American College of Neuropsychopharmacology, San Juan, Puerto Rico, December 1983

Sargant W: The treatment of anxiety states and atypical depressions by the monoamine oxidase inhibitor drugs. J Neuropsychiatry 3(Suppl 1):96–103, 1962

Schatzberg AF, Cole JO: Benzodiazepines in depressive disorders. Arch Gen Psychiatry 35:1359–1365, 1978

Schatzberg AF, Cole JO, Blumer DP: Speech blockage: a tricyclic side effect. Am J Psychiatry 135:600–601, 1978

Schatzberg AF, Rosenbaum AH, Orsulak PJ, et al: Toward a biochemical classification of depressive disorders, III: pretreatment urinary MHPG levels as predictors of response to maprotiline. Psychopharmacology 75:34–38, 1981

Schatzberg AF, Cole JO, Cohen BM, et al: Survey of depressed patients who have failed to respond to treatment, in Affective Disorders. Edited by Davis JM, Maas J. Washington, DC, American Psychiatric Press, 1983

Spiegel K, Kalb R, Pasternak GW: Analgesic activity of tricyclic antidepressants. Ann Neurol 13:462–465, 1983

Spiker DG, Hanin I, Cofsky J, et al: Pharmacological treatment of delusional depressives. Psychopharmacol Bull 17:201–202, 1981

Stark P, Fuller RW, Wong DT: The pharmacologic profile of fluoxetine. J Clin Psychiatry 46(3, sec 2):7–13, 1985

Stewart JW, Harrison W, Quitkin FM, et al: Phenelzine-induced pyridoxine deficiency. J Clin Psychopharmacol 4:225–226, 1984

Switching MAOI's [Newsnote]. Biological Therapies in Psychiatry 7(9):33–36, 1984

Tyrer P: Towards rational therapy with monoamine oxidase inhibitors. Br J Psychiatry 128:354–360, 1976

Walsh BT, Stewart JW, Wright L, et al: Treatment of bulimia with monoamine oxidase inhibitors. Am J Psychiatry 139:1629–1630, 1982

Wernicke JF: The side effect profile and safety of fluoxetine. J Clin Psychiatry 46(3, sec 2):59–67, 1985

West ED, Dally PJ: Effects of iproniazid in depressive syndromes. Br Med J 1:1491, 1959

Antipsychotic Drugs

4

In 1952, chlorpromazine was developed as an antiautonomic drug to protect the body against its own excessive compensatory reactions during major surgery. It spread into psychiatry from the field of anesthesia, after an initial clinical report by Delay et al. (1952) demonstrated the drug's good features and its efficacy in acute psychosis. Endless subsequent double-blind studies have served chiefly to confirm the effects already obvious to the original French clinicians.

In general, we are not greatly advanced from the point reached by Delay et al. in 1952, although we now know a great deal more about how antipsychotic drugs probably work and a great deal more about their side effects and about their limitations.

THE DRUGS

There are, at the time of writing, 15 antipsychotic drugs available for prescription use in the United States: nine phenothiazines, two thioxanthines, one dibenzazepine, two butyrophenones, and an indole (Table 4-A, Figure 4-1). (One of these, pimozide, is approved only for use in Gilles de la Tourette's syndrome, but it is almost certainly an effective antipsychotic.) All but three of the 15 are variants on the three-ring phenothiazine structure, and all are reasonably potent postsynaptic dopamine receptor blockers (dopamine antagonists). Although it is conceivable that these drugs might act in psychosis by some other mechanism, it seems unlikely. The only other available type of drug with some documented efficacy in schizophrenia, reserpine, presumably works to reduce dopaminergic brain activity by depleting cells of dopamine instead of blocking receptors. Only one clinically proven antipsychotic dibenzazepine—clozapine— *may* work by a different mechanism. Other drugs such as lithium carbonate and carbamazepine (see Chapter 5), pro-pranolol, diazepam, and alprazolam (see Chapter 6) have been shown to ameliorate schizophrenic symptoms under some circumstances in some patients, but none of these have clear, proven efficacy at all comparable to the standard antipsychotics.

All the effective antipsychotic drugs, except clozapine, act on the nigrostriatal system in the predicted manner, producing pseudoparkinsonism. It is presumed, but by no means proven, that the antipsychotics ameliorate schizophrenia by acting on mesolimbic or mesocortical dopamine systems. The drugs also have endocrine effects through dopamine receptors in the hypothalamic-pituitary axis. Of these, only the endocrine and nigrostriatal effects are at all helpful in understanding the clinical use of the drugs and then only in explaining and treating common side effects. As far as the major clinical action of the standard antipsychotic drugs are concerned, they could equally well be conceived to be working on the pineal gland or the psyche. Unfortunately, we do not as yet have an effective, safe antipsychotic without parkinsonian and related side effects. Even though clozapine has been known to be unique in its action on psychosis for over 10

Table 4-A. Antipsychotic Drugs

Generic Name	Brand Name	Dosage Forms
acetophenazine	Tindal	Tablets: 20 mg
chlorproma-zine	Thorazine*	Tablets: 10/25/50/100/200 mg Spansules: 30/75/150/200 mg Suppositories: 25/100 mg Syrup: 10 mg/5 ml (4 oz bottles) Concentrate: 30 mg/ml (4 oz bottles) 100 mg/ml (8 oz bottles) Ampules: 25 mg/ml (1 ml and 2 ml) Multidose vials: 25 mg/ml (10 ml)
chlorpro-thixene	Taractan	Tablets: 10/25/50/100 mg Concentrate: 100 mg/5 ml (16 oz bottles) Ampules: 25 mg/2 ml
droperidol	Inapsine	2.5 mg/ml Ampules: 2 ml and 5 ml 10 ml vials
fluphenazine HCl	Permitil	Tablets: 0.25/2.5/5/10 mg Concentrate: 5 mg/ml (4 oz bottles)
	Prolixin	Tablets: 1/2.5/5/10 mg Elixir: 2.5 mg/5 ml (16 oz bottles) Parenteral: 2.5 mg/ml (10 ml vials)
fluphenazine decanoate	Prolixin decanoate	Syringes: 25 mg/ml (1 ml) Vials: 5 ml
haloperidol	Haldol*	Tablets: 1/2/5/10 mg Concentrate: 2 mg/ml (15 ml and 120 ml bottle) Parenteral: 5 mg/ml Ampule: 1 ml Syringe (disposable): 1 ml Vial: 10 ml
loxapine	Loxitane	Capsules: 5/10/25/50 mg Concentrate: 25 mg/ml (120 ml bottle) Parenteral: 50 mg/ml Vial: 1 ml/10 ml
mesoridazine	Serentil	Tablets: 10/25/50/100 mg Concentrate: 25 mg/ml (4 oz bottles) Ampules: 25 mg/ml (1 ml)

Table 4-A. Antipsychotic Drugs (*continued*)

Generic Name	Brand Name	Dosage Forms
molindone	Moban	Tablets: 5/10/25/50/100 mg Concentrate: 20 mg/ml (120 ml bottle)
perphenazine	Trilafon	Tablets: 2/4/8/16 mg Repetabs: 8 mg Concentrate: 16 mg/5 ml (4 oz bottle) Ampules: 5 mg/ml (1 ml)
pimozide	Orap	Tablets: 2 mg
piperacetazine	Quide	Tablets: 10/25 mg
prochlorpera- zine	Compazine	Tablets: 5/10 mg Spansules: 10/15/30 mg Suppositories: 2.5/5/25 mg Syrup: 5 mg/5 ml (4 oz bottles) Parenteral: 5 mg/ml Ampules: 2 ml Syringe (disposable): 2 ml Vial: 10 ml (multidose)
thioridazine	Mellaril*	Tablets 10/15/25/50/100/150/200 mg Concentrate: 30 mg/ml, 100 mg/ml (16 oz bottles) Suspension: 25 mg/5 ml, 100 mg/5 ml (16 oz bottles)
thiothixene	Navane	Capsules: 1/2/5/10/20 mg Concentrate: 5 mg/ml (4 oz bottles) Parenteral: 2 mg/ml, 5 mg/ml Vials: 2 mg
trifluoperazine	Stelazine*	Tablets: 1/2/5/10 mg Concentrate: 10 mg/ml (2 oz bottles) Parenteral: 2 mg/ml Vials: 10 ml

*Available in generic form.

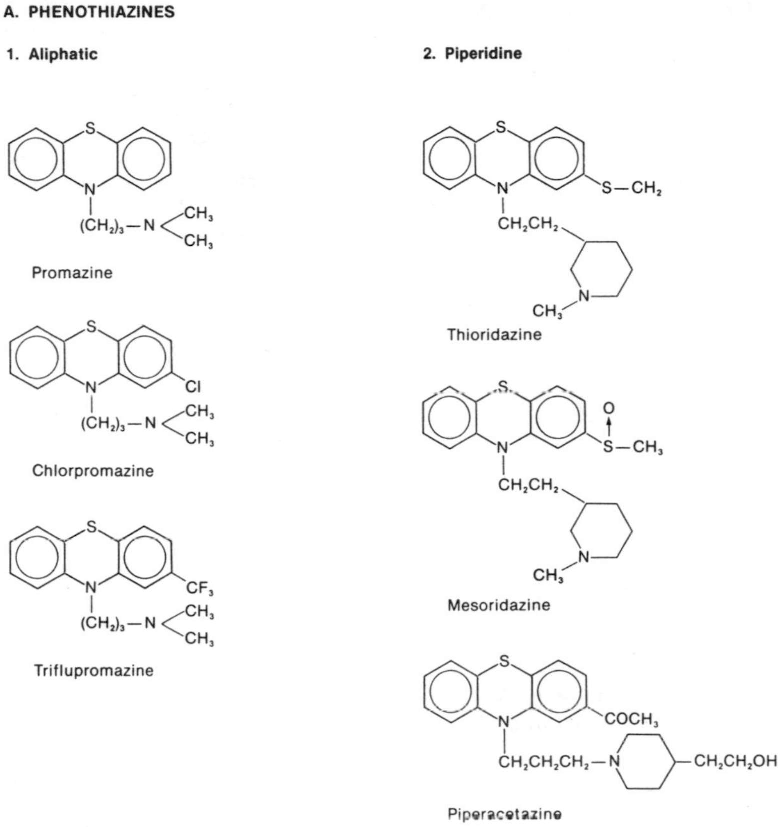

A. PHENOTHIAZINES

1. Aliphatic

Promazine

Chlorpromazine

Triflupromazine

2. Piperidine

Thioridazine

Mesoridazine

Piperacetazine

Figure 4-1. Chemical Structures of Antipsychotic Drugs

years, no comparable drug has been discovered to replace it despite the efforts of many major pharmaceutical firms. Since clozapine causes agranulocytosis and is therefore not currently available, except as an investigational drug to treat patients unable to tolerate standard antipsychotic drugs, this chapter will consider only the standard drugs.

EFFICACY

All the available standard antipsychotic drugs have been clearly shown to be more effective than placebo in schizo-

3. Piperazine

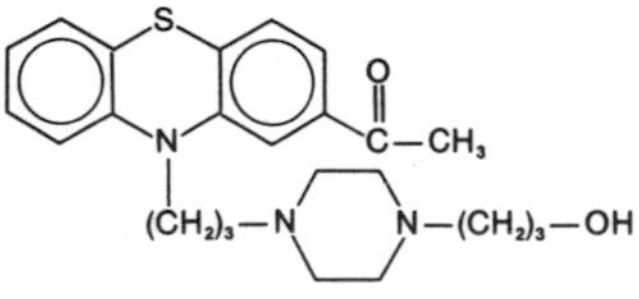

Acetophenazine

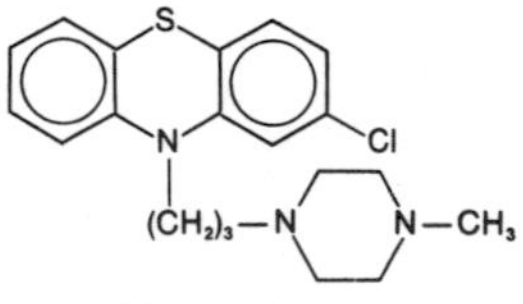

Prochlorperazine

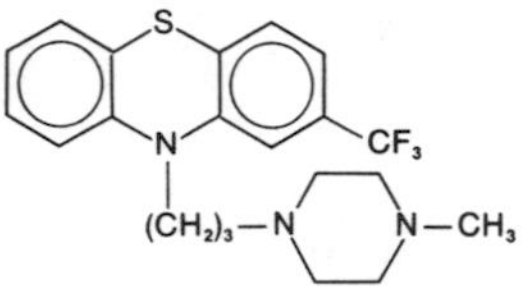

Trifluoperazine

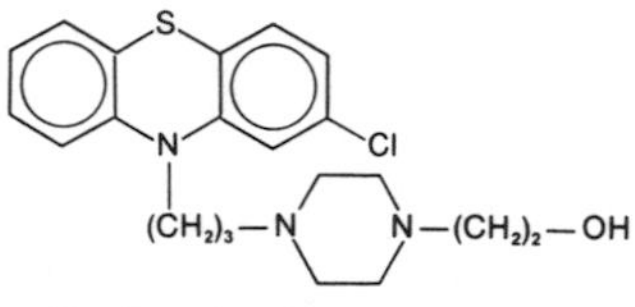

Perphenazine

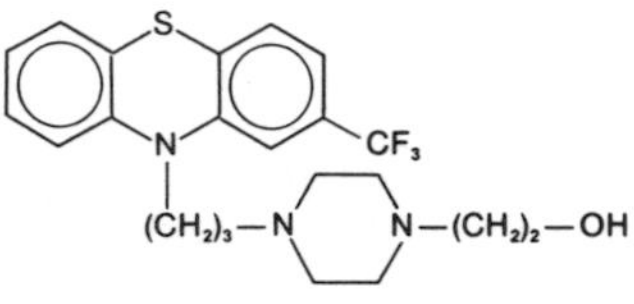

Fluphenazine

Figure 4-1. Chemical Structures of Antipsychotic Drugs (*Continued*)

phrenia, both acute and chronic. Most major studies were done many years ago using some variant of the older *DSM-II* criteria and involved an unknown but possibly large proportion of acute patients who might be judged schizophreniform or atypical bipolar or schizoaffective by current *DSM-III* standards. It is, therefore, clinically sensible to assume that all the drugs are effective in all these *DSM-III* conditions and to include mania as a proved indication as well. Since the chronic patient studies surely contained mainly *DSM-III* schizophrenic patients, there is little doubt that "real" schizophrenia responds to antipsychotic drugs as well.

B. BUTYROPHENONE-LIKE

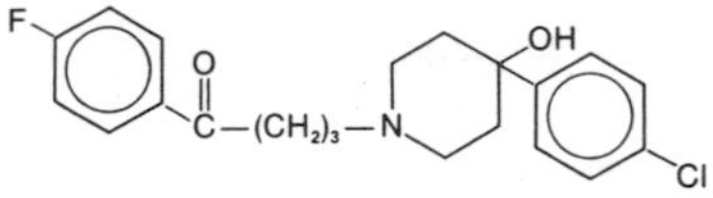

Haloperidol

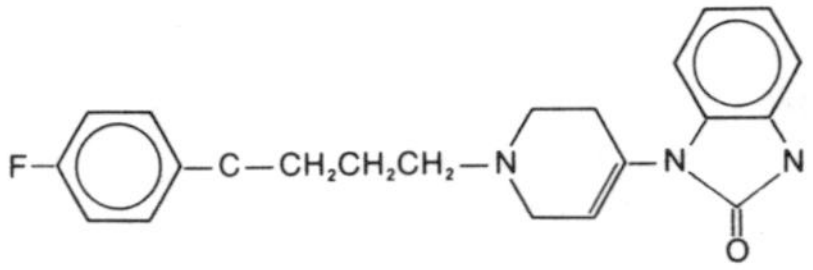

Droperidol

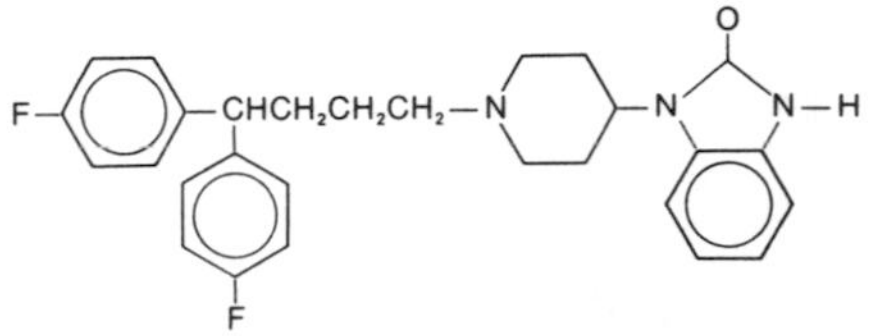

Pimozide

C. THIOXANTHENES

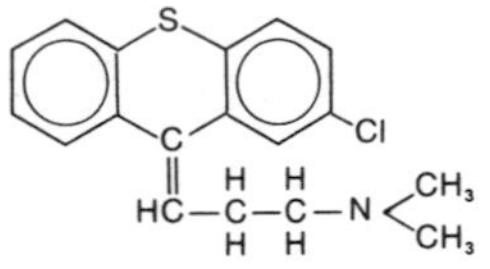

Chlorprothixene

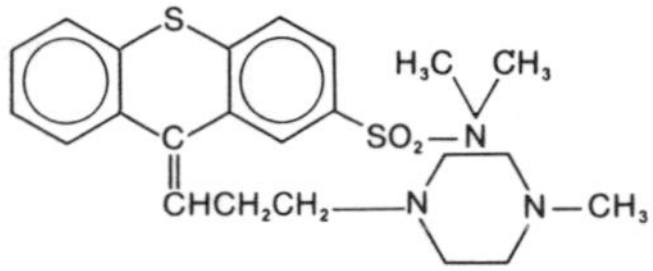

Thiothixene

Figure 4-1. Chemical Structures of Antipsychotic Drugs (*Continued*)

In many respects, the nature and timing of clinical response to antipsychotics is unsatisfactory. In large-scale six-week placebo-controlled trials in hospitalized patients, 75 percent of drug-treated patients showed at least moderate improvement, whereas only 25 percent of placebo-treated patients did as well and some got worse. However, many patients never achieve complete remission and few are able to function at a fully effective level upon return to the community.

Antipsychotic drugs are also relatively unsatisfactory as maintenance therapy. In one major study one-half of the antipsychotic-treated schizophrenic patients relapsed over the two-year study period. About 85 percent of the placebo-

D. INDOLE

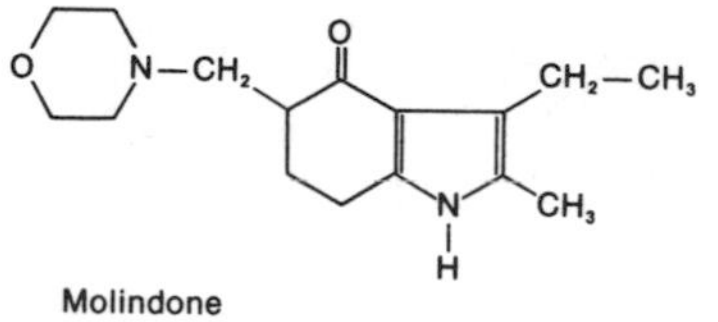

Molindone

E. DIBENZAZEPINE

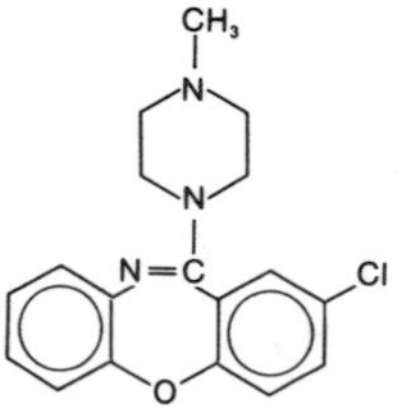

Loxapine

Figure 4-1. Chemical Structures of Antipsychotic Drugs (*Continued*)

treated patients relapsed over the same period. It thus appears that antipsychotics are more effective than placebo, but many patients relapse despite adequate drug therapy.

Further, the drugs tend to act in a slow, approximate manner. A few patients show rapid, excellent response, but most get better more slowly and some do not respond at all or only very slowly. The response is so slow and variable, sometimes, as to encourage the prescribing of very high drug dosages early in treatment in an understandable but probably misguided effort to speed clinical response.

Similarly, once a patient is better, it is almost impossible to find the minimal effective maintenance dose in any reliable way. One might imagine that the physician could gradually reduce the dose from that on which the patient had recovered (e.g., 20 mg of haloperidol a day) by 2 mg a week until psychotic symptoms began to reemerge (e.g., 6 mg a day) and then raise the dose a little until the patient is restabilized; the final dose (e.g., 8 mg a day) would then be the minimal effective maintenance dose. Unfortunately, when stable patients are shifted from an antipsychotic drug to placebo abruptly, they relapse in a leisurely and completely unpredictable rate over months and even years. There are only a few patients who relapse so rapidly that a minimum maintenance dose can actually be determined easily.

Although the available drugs differ in their side effects, both on the average and—less predictably—in individual patients, there are no obvious overall differences between the antipsychotic drugs in clinical efficacy in particular types of schizophrenic patients or in stages of illness on which to base the choice of a particular drug. The clinician can guess that an anxious, excited, acutely psychotic patient may respond better to a sedative drug like chlorpromazine, or the clinician can guess that a less sedative but less hypotensive drug like haloperidol might be better because relatively larger doses are likely to be better tolerated. Either choice is acceptable.

There is a small series of studies by Van Putten (1978) which show that if the first dose of an antipsychotic is judged even slightly helpful by a patient, that patient will have a good response to the drug over a four-week trial, whereas if the first dose is unpleasant because of oversedation or early signs of akathisia, the patient will do badly during a four-week trial even if antiparkinson drugs and dosage adjustment are used to their best advantage. (It may be—although no one has tried such an irregular approach—that one should give acutely ill patients a different drug every day until one is found that the patient does not dislike.)

The inverse of this is to take good drug histories, whenever possible, and to avoid drugs which the patient remembers to have been unpleasant.

The drugs *do* differ in the dosages and formulations in

which they are available. Thioridazine, chlorprothixene, and acetophenazine are not available in parenteral forms, and acetophenazine is only available in single (20 mg) dosage strength. Generic, and therefore less expensive, forms are now available for chlorpromazine, trifluoperazine, and thioridazine, and the patent on several others including haloperidol will be expiring shortly. So far, there is no evidence that generic forms are significantly different from the original product, but some patients will strongly prefer the old standby. Haloperidol may have a special tactical advantage in having a tasteless, colorless elixir, while chlorpromazine and thioridazine, at least, taste very medicinal. A list of available dosages and formulations is given in Table 4-A.

Only fluphenazine is available in a long-acting depot preparation in the United States, although a number of other depot drugs plus an oral tablet (penfluridol), which lasts a week, are available in Europe and, in some cases, Canada. Depot fluphenazine is available both as the enanthate and the decanoate, but there is no clear evidence that these are notably different from each other.

Since one of the main reasons antipsychotics do not work is because patients dislike them and refuse to take them, depot fluphenazine has the great advantage in that a known amount of drug is administered reliably and that the staff is immediately aware when an injection is missed. Several controlled studies have failed, however, to show that depot fluphenazine is any more effective than oral fluphenazine in averting psychotic relapse in aftercare patients. Our interpretation of these discouraging data is that research studies with dedicated nurses and excellent outreach and weekly medication monitoring, with all patients getting both pills and injections, provide an excellent but unreal level of aftercare that ensures both pill and injection taking. In more typical understaffed aftercare programs, depot fluphenazine injections will most likely be much easier to monitor and will be better monitored than pill taking. More "naturalistic"

Table 4-B. Antipsychotic Drug Potency

Generic Name	Brand Name	Chlorpromazine Equivalence
acetophenazine	Tindal	4.25
chlorpromazine	Thorazine	1.00
chlorprothixene	Taractan	2.25
clozapine	Clozaril	1.65
fluphenazine HCl	Prolixin	85.00
fluphenazine decanoate	Prolixin Decanoate	1 cc/month = 400 mg/day
haloperidol	Haldol	62.50
loxapine	Loxitane	6.65
mesoridazine	Serentil	1.80
molindone	Moban	10.00
perphenazine	Trilafon	11.25
piperactezine	Quide	9.50
prochlorperazine	Compazine	7.00
reserpine	Serpasil	66.70
thioridazine	Mellaril	1.00
thiothixene	Navane	19.20
trifluoperazine	Stelazine	35.70
triflupromazine	Vesprin	3.50

studies would have likely shown depot drug to be better at averting relapse, especially in patients with a history of noncompliance.

The next issue is the comparative potencies of the various available antipsychotics. Several experts have tried their hand at determining this. Our version is in Table 4-B.

One last general comment about antipsychotics is in order. Although we can think of only very few reasons for using two antipsychotics concurrently, there is no evidence that such a practice would be toxic or hazardous to the patient. Polypharmacy is generally frowned upon, and the use of two antipsychotics together must require a clinical justification. The only one that comes readily to mind is the use of a sedative, low-potency antipsychotic at bedtime and a high potency antipsychotic during the day in the rare patient who has insomnia on the high-potency drug alone but is oversedated if a low-potency drug is used by itself to control psychopathology.

THERAPY

Early Treatment and Crisis Intervention

Over the past few years, a great deal has been written and several small to medium-size double-blind studies have been carried out to determine how best to medicate acutely psychotic, anxious, delusional, hallucinated, angry, bizarre patients with presumptive schizophrenia, schizophreniform, or manic conditions who present in emergency rooms or are newly admitted to psychiatric wards. There are strong proponents of intensive megadose regimens such as "rapid neuroleptization," in which dosages on the order of 10 mg of haloperidol every hour or 5 mg every half hour or even a single 30 mg loading dose are given until the patient becomes calm. Probably any of the high potency drugs could be used, although only haloperidol, fluphenazine, and thiothixene have been studied systematically. Chlorpromazine used to be prescribed in such situations, but repeated dosages of 50 mg intramuscularly will cause patients to be oversedated and seriously hypotensive, whereas very large repeated doses of the high-potency drugs noted above are better tolerated (except for the side effects of dystonia and akathisia). Droperidol, marketed only for use in anesthesia, may be the most rapidly effective drug given parenterally. It is quite sedative.

It is easy to see why the clinician or ward or crisis unit staff confronted by a strikingly psychotic patient might wish to pull out all the stops in an attempt to achieve rapid reduction in psychosis. Unfortunately, the data from controlled studies, to date, show only that a very high dose (e.g., 100 mg of haloperidol or 200 mg of fluphenazine per day) has no advantage over a low dose, even in the first few hours of treatment. It is not even clear that intramuscular medication acts more rapidly than oral medication, and it is even possible, though unproved, that 2 mg of lorazepam given im may produce more rapid calming in such situations. (See reviews by both Ayd [1985] and Cole [1982].)

A conservative but effective approach is to give a moderate dose of an antipsychotic (e.g., 5 mg of haloperidol, 25 mg of loxapine, 2 mg of fluphenazine, or even 50 mg of chlorpromazine) and wait, adding a benzodiazepine if the patient continues to be overexcited after an hour or two. Intramuscular medication can be given if the patient is a danger to himself or others, but oral medication can often be used. Liquid medication is preferable because patients may cheek tablets or capsules and avoid swallowing them. The patient should be begun on a sensible, modest daily dose of an antipsychotic as indicated.

In situations of rampaging, uncontrollable, dangerous psychosis in patients who have to be held in open, nonpsychiatric facilities, restraint and more frequent larger doses may be unavoidable, but one may well be treating the situation rather than the patient. It is possible that the patients who have been enrolled in double-blind acute studies differ from those who are claimed to require crash, high-dose neuroleptization, but it is best to keep doses as low as possible under all situations.

Early Inpatient Treatment

There is no evidence that dosages higher than 15 mg of haloperidol or 400 mg of chlorpromazine a day or the equivalent are any more effective during the first few weeks of treatment than the above, reasonably standard low doses. Perhaps doses as low as 4 mg of haloperidol or 200 mg of thioridazine are, in fact, adequate. As noted above, schizophrenic patients improve relatively slowly, showing some change in the first week with further improvement up to the sixth week. This improvement can occur over a wide range of dosages. Acute controlled drug studies generally fail to find an antipsychotic dose so low that improvement does not occur, while very high doses are *less* effective than lower dosages.

The psychiatrist faced with a disturbed patient and a concerned or even frightened ward staff who are used to high neuroleptic dosages and frequent prn medication may be hard put to keep to a low, sensible, steady dosage regimen, but we strongly believe that the latter alternative is best. Again, the use of oral and parenteral benzodiazepines such as lorazepam may be more useful than giving higher dosages of neuroleptic, and they may provide more benefit to both patient and staff.

Picking the "right" drug for the patient may not be possible, and the actual drug used may often be irrelevant, all available neuroleptics being essentially equivalent in average efficacy. Nevertheless, it is well worth getting a detailed drug history from patients, family, and past physicians for patients with prior antipsychotic therapy. The point is to find out which drugs the patient has received and responded to—or those the patient has had bad reactions to or disliked actively—and to try to pick a drug that the patient will respond to.

Thioridazine should probably be avoided in sexually active younger males because of its sexual side effects, unless these patients have had akathisia or dystonia on higher potency drugs. We tend to use haloperidol, perphenazine, and loxapine more than other drugs for no documentable reason other than general personal preference. Molindone might be preferred in overweight patients because of its tendency to promote modest weight loss. As noted in Chapter 1, it is sensible to stick with a few drugs so that one becomes familiar with their dosages and idosyncracies. The only other consideration is that relapsing recurrently or chronically psychotic patients might be started on oral fluphenazine to see if it is well tolerated as an intermediate step toward shifting the patient to depot fluphenazine. Patients with insomnia that is not responsive to high-potency, low-dose neuroleptics could be shifted to chlorpromazine or chlorprothixene (100-300 mg) at bedtime for greater hypnotic effect.

If a patient actively dislikes the first few doses of a particular antipsychotic, it seems reasonable to try one or two others to see if the patient will feel less bad and cooperate more.

In the initial days of treatment, liquid medication is preferable to ensure ingestion, and doses should probably be divided with lower doses given two or three times a day and a higher dosage at bedtime. There is no clear evidence that this is any more effective than once-a-day or twice-a-day regimens, but it may make treatment induction smoother.

Similarly, the use of prn dosages in agitated patients have no proven efficacy but are often appreciated by ward staff and sometimes by patients, since they give the impression that the crisis is being managed. Perhaps prn prescription of a benzodiazepine—lorazepam at 1 or 2 mg or diazepam at 5 mg—would, in fact, give more symptomatic relief, and parenteral sodium amobarbital or lorazepam may quiet a wildly excited patient more effectively than an antipsychotic in a patient already receiving antipsychotics on a regular basis.

Some patients may become oversedated as their symptoms improve. If this occurs, the neuroleptic dose should be adjusted downward.

If a patient does not improve on an adequate dose of an antipsychotic, the choices available are several, although the reasons for selecting a specific one remain obscure. A different antipsychotic drug can be tried, of course. However, in the absence of undesirable side effects, it is always difficult to be sure whether a shift to a different drug at more or less equivalent dose will do better than continuing the original drug for a longer period. Pragmatically, two weeks without response in a markedly psychotic patient and five to six weeks in a patient with milder symptoms or with detectable but quite inadequate improvement generally forces the clinician to make a change or to add a different class of drug such as lithium. Again, the choice of the second drug is more clearly determined by the patient's past untoward reactions to specific neuroleptics than by any rational strategy based on the patient's specific pattern of psychopathology. There are, however, limited data suggesting chlorpromazine may be worth trying in badly disorganized, markedly thought-disordered patients, and loxapine may be preferred in paranoid schizophrenia (Bishop et al. 1977). Shifting chemical class sounds rational, but no one really knows whether fluphenazine resembles, say, perphenazine more than haloperidol or molindone. Some clinicians end up selecting the last drug that worked for them in a similar treatment-resistant patient.

Since patients who are failing to respond have usually already been tried on more of the original antipsychotic without benefit, it is better to use the time of change to see if a substantially lower equivalent dose of the new drug will be any better. Again, if the second drug is well tolerated, it should be continued for several weeks. The only situation in which changing drugs can be dramatic is a shift to parenteral or depot medication in a patient who has not actually been taking his or her oral medication. As Donald Klein once said, "The first thing to do when a drug isn't working is to make sure the patient is actually taking it!"

It is too early to be certain whether neuroleptic plasma levels will be of major value in titrating dose, but there are enough suggestions of the existence of a therapeutic window with some antipsychotics that plasma levels could be tried cautiously in patients who do not improve. "Therapeutic" ranges really do not exist, but laboratories can provide commonly observed blood level ranges. If a patient's blood level (12 hours after an oral dose or a week after a depot injection) is either very high or almost undetectable, then appropriate changes can be tried. If the patient is already on a very high dose of a neuroleptic and the laboratory finds almost none in the blood, one should change drugs (or laboratories) or double-check on compliance. We worry about escalating neuroleptics to huge dosages on laboratory data alone unless one has access to an outstandingly competent laboratory.

In patients who appear not to be responding to treatment, careful reevaluation of the patient for overt and covert side effects is necessary. Addition (or removal) of antiparkinsonian drugs or other medications designed to alleviate specific side effects or shifting to another neuroleptic may be helpful. Even moving the whole dose to bedtime may help by decreasing daytime sedation or inertia. Reconsidering diagnosis is also helpful. Some patients initially assumed to be schizophrenic may turn out to fit psychotic depression or atypical mania better, and the addition of an antidepressant or lithium may be positively indicated.

Some treatment-resistant *DSM-III* schizophrenic patients with little or nothing in the way of affective symptoms can improve with the addition of lithium to an antipsychotic, although this rarely results in a full remission. If a patient is unremittingly and seriously psychotic and quite probably either worse or no better on antipsychotic drugs, he needs to be tried off all antipsychotics to make sure that he is not made worse by them. Moreover, their use, in the face of little apparent response, needs to be justified because of the risk of dyskinesia.

This advice is remarkably hard to implement in many clinical situations, which is a great pity. It should also be remembered that electroconvulsive therapy *is* effective in catatonic excitements and is often helpful, at least to terminate an episode, in drug-resistant schizophrenia. It is also worth doing toxic urine screens and blood phencyclidine levels to make sure the patient is not continuing to take illicit drugs even in the hospital.

Maintenance Drug Therapy

There is no evidence as to how long to keep a patient who has recovered from a first psychotic episode on neuroleptic therapy. Probably stopping the drug two days after the patient looks much better will lead to a return of psychosis, whereas after three months many patients, perhaps 85 percent, might tolerate three weeks off medication without relapsing. At some point, the drug action seems to shift from being directly antipsychotic to preventing relapse. In principle, and generally in practice, schizophrenics reach a stable level of remission, often with residual psychotic symptoms which do not, then, improve with increased medication and even may not worsen when the drug is stopped; in fact, some patients feel "better," with more alertness and energy, off medication. However, the risk of relapse is a good deal greater off medication.

To return to the first-episode patient in full remission, prolonged antipsychotic treatment is not indicated, but it seems sensible to keep the patient on a very gradually decreasing dose of the drug on which he improved for at least three months after discharge or from the point of marked improvement. If the patient will be under predictable stress in the next six to nine months (e.g., completing school, starting a new job, getting divorced, etc.) we favor continuing the neuroleptic until that stress point is well past and the patient is generally coping adequately.

For patients with a history of three or more psychotic episodes which appear to come on after they have been taken or have taken themselves off antipsychotics, then maintenance antipsychotic therapy is indicated.

This issue is under serious question, however, and systematic large scale studies are under way which may challenge our old beliefs. At the moment, Kane's work suggests that as little as about 2.5 mg (0.1 ml) of fluphenazine decanoate every two weeks (actually 10 percent of the fluphenazine decanoate dose on which the patient has been clinically stable) is more effective than placebo in preventing relapse though less effective than the full (100 percent) dose (Kane et al. 1983). The 10 percent dose illustrates current risk-benefit problems; the patients on this dose appear to feel better, function a bit better, and are judged better by their families than patients on 100 percent dose and also develop fewer dyskinetic movements but relapse into psychosis more! Is this "better" or "worse" overall? It appears likely that a 20 percent dose (e.g., about 5 mg every 2 weeks) may be as effective as the full dose at preventing relapse.

The other option, espoused by both Carpenter and Herz, is that patients with recurring schizophrenic relapses should be followed every two to four weeks but should receive drug therapy only when and if they show symptoms of impending relapse. It is still unclear whether this option will be better or worse in terms of long-term outcome or short-term social adjustment or occurrence of tardive dyskinesia than the other two options.

At the moment, we favor stabilizing chronic relapsing schizophrenic patients in the community for three to six months, then tapering the dose very slowly over six to nine months to about 20 percent of the initial therapeutic dose, increasing the dose if psychotic or dysphoric symptoms reemerge.

Other problems in maintenance antipsychotic therapy are evident. First, maintenance only averts relapse in about half of the patients on that regimen. Second, it is often very hard to determine whether the patient relapsed because he stopped his antipsychotic medication or whether he stopped his medication because he began to relapse. Third, as tardive dyskinesia gradually emerges, the clinician gets more and more uncomfortable about continuing medication. Fourth, many chronic schizophrenics well stabilized in the community get very rigid about their treatment, and get upset (and relapse) if their medication is changed. We recently had several long-term aftercare patients who had been on neuroleptics for over five years relapse with as little as a 40 percent decrease in their antipsychotic dose.

Maintenance antipsychotic therapy in nonschizophrenic patients is *not*, generally, a good idea at all. The risk of dyskinesia is real, and the burden is on the clinician to prove that maintenance therapy was, in fact, necessary and effective. This can, of course, sometimes be the case. Trials off medication to demonstrate continued need for it are not clearly indicated in recurring chronic schizophrenia but are really required to defend maintenance neuroleptic therapy in mental retardation, affective disorders, demented elderly patients, or patients with borderline or other personality disorders.

Use in Depression

Thioridazine is approved by the Food and Drug Administration for "use" in moderate to marked depression with anxiety or agitation, and there is reasonable evidence that other neuroleptics are sometimes helpful by themselves or in combination with tricyclics or other antidepressants. However, no neuroleptic is generally superior to standard antidepressants. Because of the risk of tardive dyskinesia, neuroleptics alone or in combination should only be used in the drug therapy of depression when paranoid symptoms are present or when agitation is marked and other treatments have failed. Patients who have been on neuroleptics for typical or atypical major depressive disorders for prolonged periods are sometimes very, very difficult to wean from the neuroleptic.

Use in Anxiety

Although very low doses of neuroleptics (25 mg of chlorpromazine, 0.5 mg of haloperidol, 2 mg of trifluoperazine,

2 mg of thiothixene) given twice or three times a day or in equivalent amounts at bedtime to promote sleep are sometimes effective in generalized anxiety disorder, this regimen has not been extensively studied. As noted in Chapter 6, tricyclic antidepressants carry less risk and are probably at least as effective as antipsychotic drugs. Neuroleptics should only be used in anxiety states when more appropriate drugs fail.

Some recent studies suggest that borderline personality disorder may respond to some extent to low-dose neuroleptic therapy. Thiothixene and haloperidol have been the subjects of the only completed controlled studies which show such drugs to be superior to placebo.

Use in Organic States

Antipsychotics are widely used in agitated organic states such as delirium, senile dementia, and mental retardation with little evidence that they are really helpful. Sometimes they cause more harm through side effects than they do good, and their use is strictly empirical—valuable only if they help (see Chapter 12).

In conditions such as depression, anxiety, personality disorder, or organic brain syndromes where efficacy is not firmly established, other drug therapies or no drug therapy may be preferable.

The use of antipsychotics should *never* be routine, and their effects should always be carefully monitored and their effectiveness in each particular case documented most carefully.

SIDE EFFECTS

Sedation

Sedation, often accompanied by fatigue, can be useful early in treatment and a liability after the patient is improved. All antipsychotics can be sedative in some patients at some dose, but chlorpromazine is generally the most sedative. Its sedative effects are often judged very unpleasant by normal volunteers receiving even 25 mg or 50 mg of the drug in a single dose, but they are sometimes accepted or even welcomed by some psychotic or personality disorder patients. Thioridazine, chlorprothixene, and loxapine are also often relatively sedative, while the other high potency antipsychotics are often less sedative or not at all so. In one acute dosage strategy, the antipsychotic dosage is gradually raised until the psychosis comes under control, at which point the patient will develop increased sedation, which then requires dosage reduction.

In chronic administration, sedation and fatigue overlap with akinesia, a side effect characterized by inertia, inactivity, and lack of spontaneous movement. Akinesia will often abate when an antiparkinsonian drug is added.

When antipsychotics are used as prn medication, it is likely that sedation is the main effect produced even though decrease in psychosis may be desired. As has been discussed, a benzodiazepine (e.g., 1 or 2 mg of lorazepam) may be more appropriate for this purpose. Unfortunately, the short- (or long-) term utility of prn medication of any sort, whether as a favor to the patient or as chemical restraint, has never been seriously studied.

Autonomic Side Effects

All antipsychotics can cause postural hypotension, but this is presumed to be more common and severe with the low potency drugs, at least with chlorpromazine and thioridazine, and more dangerous in elderly or infirm patients.

Antipsychotics also have anticholinergic effects, most striking with thioridazine but also clear with chlorpromazine, mesoridazine, and trifluoperazine; they are also present but to a lesser degree with the other drugs. Dry mouth and nasal congestion can occur, as can visual blurring. When antipsychotics are combined with other anticholinergic drugs (antiparkinsonian or tricyclic antidepressant drugs) delirium or bowel stasis can occur. Constipation is a milder form of this effect.

Retrograde ejaculation is fairly common with thioridazine and can occur with other drugs in this class. This can progress to impotence. Sexual effects are worth inquiring for in patients, since patients may be upset by them but hesitate to mention them spontaneously.

Endocrine Effects

The direct effect of antipsychotic drugs is an increase in blood prolactin levels. There is a large and complex literature on this, since prolactin levels have been proposed as an alternative to measuring antipsychotic blood level directly. Attempts to use prolactin level as a guide to adequate dosage in newly hospitalized patients have not been validated to date, but one study has suggested that aftercare patients with low prolactin levels are more likely to relapse than those with higher levels.

Hyperprolactinemia can cause breast enlargement and galactorrhea in both female and male patients and may play a role in the impotence in males and the amenorrhea in female patients seen occasionally on these drugs.

Weight gain, often quite excessive, can occur on all antipsychotic drugs. It is unclear whether this is a result of increased appetite or decreased activity. Molindone is believed to be less likely to cause weight gain and even may cause modest weight loss, again for unknown reasons. Although all antipsychotics except thioridazine are good antiemetics, nausea and vomiting are sometimes seen as side effects for reasons not yet determined.

Skin and Eye Complications

A variety of kinds of allergic skin rashes can occur with antipsychotics as with all other drugs but are more common with chlorpromazine.

Chlorpromazine on prolonged high dose administration can cause pigmentation of areas exposed to the light and can cause pigment deposits in the eye, chiefly the back of the cornea and the front of the lens. These almost never affect vision and do not require regular slit lamp examinations, but patients showing an opaque pupil when a light is shined into the eye should have an ophthalmological evaluation. These deposits probably only occur with chlorpromazine but could conceivably occur with other drugs.

Retinal pigmentation occurs only with thioridazine (never reported, so far, with thioridazine's metabolite mesoridazine), and its serious and irreversible effect on vision requires that thioridazine dosage be kept at or below 800 mg a day.

Chlorpromazine often causes skin photosensitivity manifested as a severe sunburn in exposed skin areas after relatively brief (30-60 minutes) exposure to direct sunlight. Block-Out or an equivalent sun screen containing paraaminobenzoic acid, which screens out ultraviolet rays, will help avoid this effect. Other antipsychotics *may* also cause photosensitivity, and patients are generally advised to wear sun creams. Sun sensitivity can best be determined by cautious exposure to the sun in gradually increased durations. Many patients will prove to tolerate the sun normally. Chlorpromazine should be avoided in patients who are likely to spend long periods out of doors at work or for pleasure.

Other or Rare Complications

Agranulocytosis has been associated with chlorpromazine and thioridazine and could presumably occur with other antipsychotics. Its incidence is low, perhaps one case in 5000 patients treated. It usually comes on in the first three months of treatment. Monitoring for agranulocytosis does not require frequent or regular blood counts. However, patients developing a sore throat and fever in the first few months of therapy require an emergency blood count to rule out this rare but serious complication. Leukopenias in the 3000-4000 range also occur and are not generally serious.

A form of allergic obstructive hepatitis was reported relatively frequently in the early days of chlorpromazine use with an incidence of 2-3 percent, but this has been much more rarely encountered in recent years. Even when it occurred it was a relatively mild transient disorder which did not lead to hepatic necrosis or permanent liver damage. Liver problems occur so rarely with other antipsychotics as to make one believe that the occasionally abnormal liver function tests seen in patients on these drugs are due to some intercurrent, unrelated event or drug. Such abnormalities, unless progressive and severe, are not a reason for discontinuing an effective antipsychotic in a patient who needs the drug, although internists tend to blame the antipsychotic without an adequate basis when abnormal liver function tests are observed.

Seizures can also occur on antipsychotics. Only promazine (no longer used) caused them with any frequency. We know of no good data available on the comparative effects of these drugs on seizure threshold but tend to suspect loxapine and chlorpromazine as being involved in the rare neuroleptic related seizures seen at McLean Hospital and presume that the high potency drugs are less likely to cause seizures. Certainly, patients with known epilepsy who are receiving anticonvulsants often receive antipsychotics without any obvious effect on seizure frequency.

Since the neuroleptic malignant syndrome usually occurs in the context of severe parkinsonism, it will be considered with the neurological side effects.

Sudden death has been associated with antipsychotic use

in healthy young adults. The mechanisms suggested include ventricular fibrillation and aspiration of food or of vomitus during a grand mal seizure, but no clear etiology is proven. Since such deaths occurred in young psychiatric patients before antipsychotic drugs were discovered, its connection with medication remains tenuous. Over the last 30 years we have heard of more sudden deaths on thioridazine (four) than on any other neuroleptic, but even these are so very rare as to make suspicion probably unwarranted.

Neurological Side Effects

Although dopamine blockade in the striatum is the most popular mechanism invoked for all neurological side effects from antipsychotic drugs and anticholinergic antiparkinsonian drugs are the conventional remedy, the presumed cholinergic/dopaminergic imbalance is probably only a partial explanation.

Dystonia. The earliest side effect, dystonia, often manifested by tonic muscle spasm in the tongue, jaw, and neck, usually occurs in the first few hours or days on an antipsychotic. It can present as a very frightening opisthotonus of the whole body with extensor rigidity or as only mild tongue stiffness. In one small study it appeared as neuroleptic blood levels were dropping, not rising, making one wonder whether it might be a rebound effect as dopamine blockade is waning. In any event, it can be fairly effectively averted by prophylactic antiparkinsonian usage (Table 4-C) and rarely occurs with thioridazine. It is more common in younger males but can occur in either sex at any age. Once present, it can be rapidly relieved by intravenous antiparkinsonian drugs (only diphenhydramine and biperiden are readily available for intravenous use) or, less rapidly, by intramuscular medication. However, such diverse drugs as diazepam, amobarbital, and caffeine

Table 4-C.   Antiparkinsonian Drugs

Generic Name	Brand Name	Formulations	Dosage Ranges (mg/day)
Primarily Anticholinergic			
benztropine	Cogentin	Tablets: 1/2 mg Parenteral: 1 mg/ml (2 ml ampule)	2–6
biperiden	Akineton	Tablets: 2 mg Parenteral: 5 mg/ml (1 ml ampule)	2–8
diphenhydramine	Benadryl	Capsules: 25/50 mg Elixir: 12.5 mg/5 ml (4 oz, 16 oz bottles) Parenteral: 10 mg/ml (10 ml, 30 ml vials) 1 ml ampule	50–300
ethopropazine	Parsidol	Tablets: 10/50 mg	100–400
procyclidine	Kemadrin	Tablets: 5 mg	10–20
trihexyphenidyl	Artane	Tablets: 2/5 mg Sequels: 5 mg capsules	4–15
Dopaminergic			
amantadine	Symmetrel	Capsules: 100 mg Syrup: 50 mg/ 5 ml (16 oz bottles)	100–300

sodium benzoate and even hypnosis have been said to relieve it as well.

Once the dystonia has resolved and the patient is protected by oral antiparkinsonian medication, the offending antipsychotic can be continued without recurrence of the dystonia, but patients often feel less apprehensive if a different antipsychotic drug is substituted. Some patients on depot fluphenazine will develop recurrences of dystonia with some succeeding injections.

Oculogyric crises, manifested by forced eye rotation, usually upward, are conventionally classified with the dystonias but can occur, even recur fairly frequently, later in treatment when more conventional dystonia is rare.

Pseudoparkinsonism.   Some time in the early stages of treatment, usually between five days and four weeks, the patient can develop signs of parkinsonism. In contrast to idiopathic Parkinson's disease, pill-rolling tremor is very rare, but muscle stiffness, cog-wheel rigidity, stooped posture, masklike facies, and even drooling are quite common. Micrographia occurs and can help differentiate antipsychotic tremor from lithium tremor.

Patients rarely develop such severe rigidity as to be incapacitated or even immobilized. When they do, such patients are sometimes misdiagnosed as having catatonia. Patients with such severe rigidity do not respond readily to even massive doses of antiparkinsonian drugs; the condition may require as long as two weeks to clear after the antipsychotic drug is stopped.

Milder degrees of pseudoparkinsonism are often seen for prolonged periods in patients on long-term maintenance medication and can contribute to passive inactivity in such patients.

Akinesia—reduction in spontaneous or voluntary movement—can be seen in patients on maintenance antipsychotic medication in the absence of signs of Parkinsonism; regular coarse tremor can also be seen alone without any other parkinsonian signs. Both conditions respond either to anti-parkinsonian drugs or reduction in neuroleptic dose.

Akathisia. This inner-driven restlessness caused by anti-psychotics is the least understood and most troublesome of their neurological side effects. It ranges from an unpleasant subjective feeling of muscular discomfort to an agitated, desperate, markedly dysphoric pacing with hand-wringing and weeping. In between these extremes, patients will find themselves unable to sit still for long, having to stand up and move about or continually shift their position. It is sometimes mistaken for psychotic agitation and treated inappropriately by an increase in antipsychotic dose. It can be experienced even after the first dose of a neuroleptic but can become a clinical problem at anytime in the first few weeks on medication. It occurs on thioridazine as well as on the more potent drugs. It is less responsive to antiparkinsonian drugs than other neurological side effects and is the bane of maintenance medication, being a common basis for patients refusing to stay on such a regimen. Recent pilot studies suggest that propranolol in doses from 30 to 120 mg a day sometimes suppresses akathisia when neither antiparkinsonian drugs nor benzodiazepines such as lorazepam work. But it is too early to tell whether propranolol will become a preferred treatment. Its presumed efficacy casts some doubt on dopamine-blockade being the mechanism underlying akathisia.

Regular rhythmic leg-jiggling up and down, or less commonly to and fro, is often seen in patients treated with antipsychotics and is probably, but not certainly, a variant of akathisia, although some consider it a form of tremor. Patients with this phenomenon are often unaware of it or not bothered by it. The best basis for differential diagnosis of akathisia is to ask the patient whether his restlessness is a "muscle" feeling or a "head" feeling—the former being akathisia and the latter, anxiety. In case of doubt, it is safer to assume akathisia exists since overdosage with neuroleptics is vastly more common than underdosage.

Use of Antiparkinsonian Drugs

For decades there have been impassioned arguments pro and con about the prophylactic use of antiparkinsonian drugs. Many senior clinicians claim that patient drug acceptance is enhanced and unpleasant side effects are averted by routine antiparkinsonian administration to all patients being started (or restarted) on antipsychotic drugs. Others, however, assert that two drugs (an antipsychotic drug plus an antiparkinsonian drug) can be more toxic than an antipsychotic alone and that an antiparkinsonian drug should only be added when neurological side effects appear. Personally, we believe there is enough evidence that antiparkinsonian drugs avert neurological side effects to use them routinely in most acutely psychotic patients under age 45 being started on a neuroleptic unless their anticholinergic side effects are contraindicated. In the less common situation in which very low, cautious trials on antipsychotics (e.g., 1-3 mg of haloperidol a day) are undertaken in mildly or nonpsychotic patients, antiparkinsonian drugs are unnecessary. If routine antiparkinsonian medication is not used prophylactically in acute patients, prn orders for such patients should be written.

After four weeks to six months of long-term maintenance antipsychotic therapy, the antiparkinsonian drugs can be shifted to prn or withdrawn. A few patients (~15 percent) will redevelop clear neurological side effects and even more (~30 percent) will feel "better"—less anxious or depressed or inert—on continued antiparkinsonian drugs. Some chronic schizophrenics are delighted to stop their neuroleptic but demand to continue their antiparkinsonian drug (Wojcik 1979). Very rarely, patients use trihexyphenidyl or other antiparkinsonians to get "high," but far more patients do better on these drugs than off them.

There are rare patients who develop anticholinergic deliria or intestinal stasis on these drugs; dry mouth and blurred vision are more common side effects. Dosage ranges of the available antiparkinsonian drugs are given in Table 4-C. Probably, if blood level determinations of either the drug itself or of anticholinergic levels by radioreceptor assay were generally available, dosage might be adjusted more rationally. At present, if a patient has neither relief of neurological side effects nor dry mouth, a cautious increase in dose—even over the maximum recommended in *PDR*—can be considered, although decreasing the neuroleptic dose may be even more rational.

Most of the antiparkinsonian drugs are assumed to work by their anticholinergic effects and are probably equivalent to one another, although we have seen rare syndromes which respond uniquely to the anticholinergic antihistamine diphenhydramine or to ethopropazine. No controlled comparative studies of these drugs exist to guide the clinician. Probably diphenhydramine is more sedative, trihexyphenidyl slightly more stimulating, and biperiden more neutral in this dimension.

Amantadine, which is presumed to work as a dopamine agonist, can be used at dosages of 200-300 mg a day. It is probably as effective as the anticholinergic antiparkinsonian drugs but has no proven advantages. Tolerance to its antiparkinsonian effects may also be more of a problem. However, it may be useful in galactorrhea by reducing blood prolactin levels. Although one might expect a dopamine agonist to be stimulant, patients sometimes find amantadine to be sedative. L-Dopa has not been systematically studied in pseudoparkinsonism. It probably works too slowly and can sometimes aggravate psychosis. The standard antiparkinsonian drugs generally have no obvious effect on the psychosis; the few controlled studies comparing antipsychotic drugs with and without added antiparkinsonian agents are equivocal.

TARDIVE DYSKINESIA

Some patients exposed to antipsychotic drugs develop abnormal, involuntary, irregular, choreiform and/or athetoid movements. These most commonly include tongue overactivity—darting, writhing, twisting, or repeated protrusions—and finger movements—choreiform or hand clenching. Chewing or lateral jaw movements, lip puckering, facial grimacing, torticollis or retrocollis, trunk twisting, pelvic thrusting, respiratory grunting, athetoid arm and shoulder movements, or a variety of toe, ankle, and leg movements all occur in a variety of combinations. These are hard to distinguish, at times, from schizophrenic mannerisms and essentially impossible to distinguish on phenomenology alone from other, rarer causes of dyskinesia. Sometimes patients show tardive dystonia instead, a variant of tardive dyskinesia with large athetoid movements of arms, face, neck, etc., ending in fixed dystonic postures which are held for 10 to 30 seconds as against the more rapid movements that are more common in ordinary tardive dyskinesia.

The severity of tardive dyskinesia ranges from minimal tongue restlessness and finger movement to gross, incapacitating disfiguring movements. Most identifiable cases are mild and not noticed by either patient or the family or passed off as minor tics or restlessness by both. Even clearly visible dyskinesias are often of little real consequence, but about 3 percent of cases are sufficiently severe to cause social or functional problems. Most patients and families seen in the Tardive Dyskinesia Clinic at McLean Hospital are much more concerned about the possible ultimate consequences of currently very mild dyskinesia than about the minor movements the patient is showing at the time of consultation.

It is currently impossible to predict which patients will develop dyskinesia, early or late, mild or severe. However, the best available data suggest a rate of development of dyskinesia of about 3-4 percent per year over the first four or five years of exposure and that elderly women and patients with affective disorders may be at the greatest risk (Gardos and Casey 1984). In chronically institutionalized psychotic patients, dyskinesia prevalence rates are often on the order of 50-60 percent.

At the extremes, a few patients develop persistent dyskinesia after only a few weeks of exposure to antipsychotics, but up to six months on antipsychotics is generally considered safe. Some patients only show dyskinesia when the neuroleptic is stopped (covert dyskinesia), whereas some who develop dyskinesia have it fade away when antipsychotics are stopped weeks, months, or years later. There is a significant rate of occurrence of dyskinesia in individuals never exposed to neuroleptics, from 1 to 5 percent, increasing with advancing age so that not all dyskinesia in patients on neuroleptics is due to the drug. Unfortunately, no one can tell which cases are idiopathic. There are no strong, consistent treatment factors related to dyskinesia, either. Duration of antipsychotic treatment correlates more commonly with dyskinesia than does total dose. There is no clear evidence that any one antipsychotic is less commonly related to tardive dyskinesia development than any other.

Basic research data on dopamine receptor overproliferation caused by neuroleptics in laboratory animals have been used to claim that drugs such as thioridazine or molindone *should* be less likely to cause tardive dyskinesia than other antipsychotics, but we have seen a number of cases in patients only or almost only exposed to thioridazine and one case on molindone. Neither periods off neuroleptics nor use of antiparkinsonian drugs seem generally related to tardive dyskinesia development. Thus, until some new, different, and safer antipsychotic emerges, there is no way to avoid tardive dyskinesia except to avoid using antipsychotics.

This means that the clinician must seriously consider the risks and benefits of extended treatment with antipsychotics in all patients likely to be kept on medication for longer than six months. This issue must be discussed with the patient and his or her family unless there are defensible clinical reasons for not doing so. Either way, everything should be documented in the patient's chart, and the process should be redone if signs of dyskinesia are noted. (See Chapter 1 for further discussion.)

To date, the available long-term (two- to 10-year) follow-up studies suggest that tardive dyskinesia is not generally a progressive disorder. In chronically psychotic patients, the best clinical decision is often to continue the antipsychotic, but this decision must be based on the available facts in each case.

There is no effective or standard treatment for tardive dyskinesia. Trying to slowly taper the antipsychotic dose is often recommended. Lithium is often added and the use of reserpine has its advocates. Also, a shift to a different antipsychotic is sometimes suggested.

Unfortunately, tardive dyskinesia is a remarkably heterogeneous condition in terms of its response to drug therapies. Although the condition is often assumed to be due to dopaminergic overactivity and should therefore be suppressed by dopamine blocking agents and aggravated by anticholinergic antiparkinsonian drugs, some patients show exactly the opposite responses, and pseudoparkinsonism paradoxically often coexists with dyskinesia. Benzodiazepines often mildly alleviate dyskinetic movements. A vast range of other centrally active drugs have been tried and sometimes have helped.

Luckily, most cases of dyskinesia are not serious enough to require or warrant special treatment to suppress the dyskinesia.

NEUROLEPTIC MALIGNANT SYNDROME

This occasionally fatal and always serious syndrome is manifested by a variable combination of symptoms and signs. These include hyperpyrexia up to 107 F and severe parkinsonian muscle rigidity with elevated creatinine phosphokinase blood levels and elevated white blood count. Consciousness is usually altered but may be obtunded or agitated. The dystonia and rigidity may be so severe as to make walking or talking difficult or almost impossible. Pulse is elevated and blood pressure is either high or low with diastolic hypertension common. Liver enzymes are usually elevated. Myoglobin in plasma may cause renal shutdown. Profuse sweating is common.

The drug treatment prior to neuroleptic malignant syndrome is very variable. It can occur in patients on a stable antipsychotic dose for months or come on suddenly when medication is being started. Symptoms usually persist for 10 to 14 days or longer in patients on short-acting antipsychotics and for four weeks or longer after depot fluphenazine.

It is hard to tell whether neuroleptic malignant syndrome is a more severe variant of severe pseudoparkinsonism seen early in drug therapy in some patients, a variant of heat stroke seen in psychiatric patients on and off antipsychotics, a result of an intercurrent viral infection, or a sequel of epileptic seizures. Gelenberg et al. have described another syndrome of catatonia in response to neuroleptics which seems to differ from pseudoparkinsonism mainly in showing waxy flexibility, posturing, and mutism but no fever or other autonomic changes.

Treatment of neuroleptic malignant syndrome is symptomatic (cooling the body to reduce fever); dantrolene (e.g., 200 mg a day) has been used to decrease muscle spasm with some success in lowering fever and tachycardia. Bromocriptine from 5 mg every four hours to 60 mg a day has been used with more rapid benefit. Regular anticholinergic antiparkinsonian drugs have not been helpful and were often already being given when the syndrome developed. Amantadine has usually not worked, but no more than 100 mg TID has been tried. There is a case of neuroleptic malignant syndrome developing when amantadine was stopped, suggesting that it might help at some dose. Generally, patients with the syndrome require careful medication titration and monitoring for four to five weeks, since the syndrome can recur even weeks after the neuroleptic has been stopped.

Almost all reported cases occurred in patients on high potency neuroleptics, so cautious retreatment with thioridazine is probably safest after the syndrome has been absent for at least two weeks, although one case has been reported on thioridazine.

ALTERNATIVES TO NEUROLEPTIC THERAPY

There are currently no reliable, safe, and effective drug therapies for schizophrenic disorders that can replace standard dopamine-blocking neuroleptics.

Electroconvulsive therapy can reverse psychotic excitements and catatonic stupor but has no real value in preventing future episodes of psychosis. Reserpine has a weak antipsychotic effect which is slow in onset; even at 10-15 mg a day, major improvement may be delayed for two months and schizophrenic patients may pass through a stage of behavioral turbulence before improving. Such a prospect is clinically discouraging, to say the least. Worse, a few early cases of dyskinesia were induced by reserpine. Lithium can ameliorate schizophrenic symptoms or suppress episodic violence in schizophrenic patients, but it almost never is an adequate drug therapy by itself. Carbamazepine also ameliorates symptoms in some treatment-resistant psychotic patients, as a double-blind Israeli study shows (Klein et al. 1984), but it is not, by itself, an adequate therapy for schizophrenia.

Recently, diazepam alone has been reported by both

Canadian and German groups to rapidly control psychotic symptoms in small numbers of paranoid schizophrenic patients at doses between 70 and 400 mg a day (the German group used 50 mg tablets). Sedation was *not* a problem, allegedly, after the first day, and improvement continued for four weeks. Neither study reported follow-up data. In one study, high-dose diazepam aggravated schizoaffective symptoms. These little, brief studies are intriguing but do not offer a real and useful pharmacological alternative to the standard antipsychotics.

Propranolol has been studied for many years in the treatment of acute and chronic schizophrenia in very high dosages (600-2000 mg a day) given alone or with a neuroleptic drug. Although Yorkston has reported efficacy in controlled studies, other investigators have found equivocal results with only occasional patients showing any benefit. Since two deaths have occurred on this treatment, one of a silent bleeding peptic ulcer and one sudden death of unknown etiology, this use cannot be generally recommended. However, more recent clinical studies of doses up to 400 mg a day in organically impaired psychiatric patients with impulsive violence or aggression suggest that propranolol may be useful in such patients in controlling temper outbursts although it does not affect the other underlying behavioral organic deficits.

If such therapy were to be attempted, the relevant articles should be reviewed and dosage increased slowly, with blood pressure and pulse monitoring before each dose until the patient is well stabilized at a constant, effective dose. Propranolol has been reported to increase chlorpromazine blood levels and may do so for other antipsychotics as well.

It is possible that carbamazepine and lithium also offer more promise in the treatment of disturbed behavior in brain damaged, demented, or mentally retarded patients than do the standard antipsychotics, but it is too early to make specific claims or recommendations in these areas. It *is* possible to assert that clinicians who use standard antipsychotics in such

nonschizophrenic patients are at risk for criticism or possibly
for a malpractice suit if they cannot convincingly document
the rationale on which the drug use is based and if they
cannot document that the antipsychotic was, in fact, clinically
useful in the particular patient treated.

Bibliography

Ayd F: Lorazepam update: 1977–1985. International Drug Therapy
    Newsletter 20:33–36, 1985

Baldessarini RJ, Cole JO, Davis JM, et al: Tardive Dyskinesia [Task
    Force Report no 18]. Washington, DC, American Psychiatric
    Association, 1980

Bishop M, Simpson G, Dunnett C, et al: Efficacy of loxapine in
    the treatment of paranoid schizophrenia. Psychopharmacology
    51:107–114, 1977

Blackwell B: Patient compliance with drug therapy. N Engl J Med
    289:249–252, 1973

Brown W, Laughren T: Low serum prolactin and early relapse
    following neuroleptic withdrawal. Am J Psychiatry 138:237–
    239, 1981

Carpenter W, Heinrichs D: Early intervention, time-limited targeted
    pharmacotherapy of schizophrenia. Schizophr Bull 9:533–542,
    1983

Cohen BM: The clinical utility of plasma neuroleptic levels, in
    Guidelines for the Use of Psychotropic Drugs. Edited by Stancer
    H. New York, Spectrum Publications, 1984, pp 245–260

Cole JO: Antipsychotic drugs: is more better? McLean Hospital
    Journal 7:61–87, 1982

Cole JO, Gardos G, Gelernter J, et al: Supersensitivity psychosis.
    McLean Hospital Journal 9:46–72, 1984

Cole JO, Gardos G: Alternatives to neuroleptic drug therapy.
    McLean Hospital Journal 10:112–127, 1985

Creese I: Dopamine and antipsychotic medications, in Psychiatry
    Update, vol 4. Edited by Hales R, Frances A. Washington,
    DC, American Psychiatric Press, 1985, pp 17–36

Davis JM: Overview: Maintenance therapy in psychiatry, I: Schiz-
    ophrenia. Am J Psychiatry 132:1237–1245, 1975

Delay J, Deniker P, Harl J: Utilization therapeutique psychiatrique d'une phenothiazine d'action centrale elective (4560 RP). Ann Med Psychol (Paris) 110:112–117, 1952

Delva N, Letemendia F: Lithium treatment in schizophrenic and schizoaffective disorders. Br J Psychiatry 141:387–400, 1982

Donaldson SR, Gelenberg AJ, Baldessarini RJ: The pharmacological treatment of schizophrenia: a progress report. Schizophr Bull 9:504–527, 1983

Finnerty RJ, Goldberg HL, Nathan L, et al: Haloperidol in neurotic outpatients. Diseases of the Nervous System 37:621–624, 1976

Galbrecht CR, Klett CJ: Predicting response to phenothiazines: the right drug for the right patient. J Nerv Ment Dis 147:173–183, 1968

Gardos G, Perenyi A, Cole J: Polypharmacy revisited. McLean Hospital Journal 5:178–195, 1980

Gardos G, Casey D: Tardive dyskinesia and affective disorders. Washington, DC, American Psychiatric Press, 1984

Gelenberg H, Mandel M: Catatonic reactions to high potency neuroleptic drugs. Arch Gen Psychiatry 34:947–952, 1977

Greendyke R, Schuster D, Wooten J: Propranolol in the treatment of assaultive patients with organic brain disease. J Clin Psychopharmacol 4:282–285, 1984

Hayes P, Schulz C: The use of beta-adrenergic blocking drugs in anxiety disorders and schizophrenia. Pharmacotherapy 3:101–117, 1983

Herz M, Szymanski H, Simon J: Intermittant medication for stable schizophrenic outpatients. Am J Psychiatry 139:918–922, 1982

Hogarty G: Treatment and course of schizophrenia. Schizophr Bull 3:587–599, 1977

Hogarty GE, Ulrich RJ: Temporal effects of drugs and placebo in delaying relapse in schizophrenic outpatients. Arch Gen Psychiatry 34:297–301, 1977

Jefferson J, Greist J: Haloperidol and lithium: their combined use and the issue of their compatability, in Haloperidol Update, 1958–1980. Edited by Ayd F. Baltimore, Ayd Medical Communications, 1980, pp 73–28

Kane JM, Rifkin A, Woerner M, et al: Low dose neuroleptic treatment of outpatient schizophrenics. Arch Gen Psychiatry 40:896, 1983

Kane J, Woerner M. Weinhold P, et al: A prospective study of tardive dyskinesia: preliminary results. J Clin Psychopharm 2:345–349, 1982

Keepers GA, Clappison VJ, Casey DE: Initial anticholinergic prophylaxis for neuroleptic-induced extrapyramidal syndromes. Arch Gen Psychiatry 40:113, 1983

Klein E, Bental E, Lerer B, et al: Carbamazepine and haloperidol v placebo and haloperidol in excited psychosis. Arch Gen Psychiatry 41:165–172, 1984

Levenson J: Neuroleptic malignant syndrome. Am J Psychiatry 142:1137–1145, 1985

Lipinski JF, Zubenko G, Cohen BM, et al: Propranolol in the treatment of neuroleptic-induced akathisia. Am J Psychiatry 141:412–415, 1984

Mason AS, Granacher RP: Clinical Handbook of Antipsychotic Drug Therapy. New York, Brunner/Mazel, 1978

May PRA: Treatment of schizophrenia: A comparative study of five treatment methods. New York, Science House, 1968

Pisciotta AV: Agranulocytosis induced by certain phenothiazine derivatives JAMA 208:1862–1868, 1969

Roy-Byrne P, Gerner R, Liston E, et al: ECT for acute mania: a forgotten treatment modality. Journal of Psychiatric Treatment and Evaluation 3:83–86, 1981

Silver J, Yudofsky S: Propranolol for aggression: literature review and clinical guidelines. International Drug Therapy Newsletter 20:9–12, 1985

Tuason V, Escobar J, Garvey M, et al: Loxapine vs chlorpromazine in paranoid schizophrenia. J Clin Psychiatry 45:158–163, 1984

Van Putten T: Why do schizophrenic patients refuse to take their drugs? Arch Gen Psychiatry 31:67–72, 1978

Wojcik J: Antiparkinson drug use. Biological Therapies in Psychiatry Newsletter 2:5–7, 1979

Yorkston N, Zaki S, Havard C: Some practical aspects of using propranolol in the treatment of schizophrenia, in Propranolol and Schizophrenia. Edited by Roberts E, Amacher P. New York, Liss, 1978, pp 83–97

Mood Stabilizers

5

The term "mood stabilizer" was first applied to the lithium salts when it became clear that these compounds not only were effective in manic excitement but also tended to avert both manic and depressive recurrences in bipolar patients. More recently, several anticonvulsants—carbamazepine, valproic acid, and probably clonazepam—have been shown to be effective in the treatment of manic excitement and may have longer term mood-stabilizing effects in some bipolar or schizoaffective patients. This chapter will consider the properties of lithium salts first and then the use of anticonvulsants in bipolar and related disorders.

LITHIUM

History and Indications

Lithium, usually as the carbonate and occasionally as the citrate salt, is widely used in American psychiatry, particularly considering that its only FDA approved indications are for

the treatment of mania and as maintenance therapy to prever
or diminish the intensity of "subsequent episodes in thos
manic-depressive patients with a history of mania." As wi
be discussed below, lithium is often used in patients with
variety of recurrent episodic illnesses with or without pron
inent affective features. It is also used in patients with moo
lability, with impulsive or episodic violence or anger, or eve
with paramenstrual dysphoria, alcoholism, borderline pe
sonality disorder, and almost any other condition that doe
not respond to other drug therapies.

The use of lithium salts in psychiatry was initiated by Joh
Cade (an Australian state hospital superintendent) in th
1940s for ultimately irrelevant reasons, but it proved to b
an effective though toxic treatment. The addition of serur
level monitoring made the treatment safe and provided th
first general use of blood level monitoring for a psychiatri
drug. The use of lithium in psychiatry generally increase
worldwide, although the United States was slow to participat
because of an earlier disastrous experience in this countr
with the unmonitored use of lithium chloride as a sa
substitute, which had led to severe toxic reactions, som
fatal.

Schou was the first to report compelling evidence that th
use of lithium carbonate reduced the incidence and duratio
of serious affective episodes dramatically in bipolar patient:
Since that time, a large number of controlled, double-blin
studies have confirmed that lithium is clearly effective i
reducing recurrences in both bipolar and unipolar affectiv
disorders, as well as being more effective than placebo i
acute mania.

Preparations

Lithium is available in the United States in several for
mulations (Table 5-A). The standard and least expensiv
format is the carbonate in 300 mg capsules or scored tablet:

Table 5-A. Mood Stabilizers

Generic Name	Brand Name	Formulations
lithium carbonate	Eskalith	300 mg tablets
		300 mg capsules
	Lithane	300 mg tablets
	Lithotabs	300 mg tablets
	Eskalith CR (sustained release)	450 mg tablets
	Lithobid (sustained release)	300 mg tablets
lithium citrate	Cibalith-S	8 mEq/5 ml (480 ml bottles)
carbamazepine	Tegretol	200 mg tablets
		100 mg chewable tablets
valproic acid	Depakene	250 mg capsules
		250 mg/5 ml (16 oz bottles)
	Depakote	125/250/500 mg enteric coated tablets
clonazepam	Klonopin	0.5/1.0/2.0 mg tablets

Sustained release preparations of the carbonate are also available as well as a liquid preparation of lithium citrate; in the latter case, one teaspoonful is the equivalent of the ion content of 300 mg of the carbonate (8 mEq). Other preparations, including the sulfate, and other dosage strengths are used in Europe. Despite over 30 years of clinical experience with lithium, it is not entirely clear whether any of the formulations have clear superiority for any purpose except that the citrate is obviously useful in patients who dislike or cannot swallow pills.

The sustained release preparations result in lower peak serum lithium levels after ingestion and probably result in less lithium ion being released in the stomach and more in the small intestine. If lithium irritation of the stomach mucosa is causing nausea after each dose, then the sustained release preparation might reduce gastric irritation. If diarrhea is a problem (and is not due to an elevated serum lithium level), then the citrate might cause even faster absorption in the upper gastrointestinal tract and might reduce the diarrhea. However, we have seen patients with diarrhea on standard lithium carbonate whose diarrhea lessened on sustained release lithium.

The basic problem is that it is still unclear which lithium side effects are related to peak serum level and which to steady state serum level. Clinically, any side effect that mainly occurs one to two hours after each oral dose of the standard preparation might be improved by the sustained release form. For example, nausea may be caused by lithium's gastric irritation or by an elevated serum level. The former would cause transient nausea after each dose; the latter would cause persistent nausea.

There was a belief that sustained release lithium would, in general, cause fewer side effects and might cause, in particular, less effect on the concentrating ability of the renal tubules, leading to less polyuria and polydipsia. So far, this does not seem to be the case and it may even be that massing the total lithium daily dose at bedtime may cause fewer renal effects. One major European center (Copenhagen) routinely has been using once a day lithium dosage for many years, suggesting that this dosage scheme is feasible and effective.

As will be noted below, sometimes lithium causes skin rashes that appear to be allergic in nature; these may be due to other ingredients in a particular lithium preparation and may disappear if a different preparation is substituted.

Blood Levels

Lithium dosage is titrated to achieve both therapeutic response and "adequate" blood levels. The general presumption is that levels of around 0.7-1.0 mEq/L are appropriate for maintenance therapy or the treatment of conditions other than manic or psychotic excitement, whereas levels up to 1.5

mEq/L are needed in acute mania. Levels should be obtained about 12 hours after the last dose, at which time the vagaries of absorption after drug ingestion are well past and a relative steady state has been achieved (see the section on Tricyclic Blood Levels in Chapter 3). These "ideal" levels are, of course, not carved in stone and must be interpreted in the clinical context. Someone who has marked tremor, oversedation, vomiting, and ataxia at a level of 0.8 mEq/L either cannot tolerate that level or has some other medical condition causing the symptoms, with lithium intolerance being the more likely. Other patients on maintenance therapy appear to have affective episodes averted for years at levels as low as 0.4 to 0.6 mEq/L, and patients with daily symptoms such as irritability and anger claim clinical improvement at very low blood levels. It is very hard to prove that these are (or are not) "real" drug responses. It is our belief that many patients can be successfully maintained at relatively low serum levels. Occasionally, a patient whose mania is still uncontrolled despite a level of 1.5 mEq/L for several days and has no side effects could be cautiously tried at a higher level.

Clinical Use Patterns

Lithium use can be divided into four general clinical contexts:

1. to control rapidly acute, overt psychopathology as in mania or psychotic agitation;
2. to attempt to modify milder ongoing or frequent but episodic clinical symptoms such as chronic depression or episodic irritability;
3. to establish a prophylactic maintenance regimen to avert future affective or psychotic episodes; or
4. to enhance the effect of antidepressants in patients with major depressive disorder (see Chapters 3 and 9).

Acute Psychosis

Here rapid establishment of high, adequate lithium levels (e.g., 1.0 to 1.5 mEq/L) is desired, and an initial regimen of 300 mg two to four times a day is indicated in healthy adolescent or adult patients with lithium serum levels obtained every one or two days. The dose is titrated up (or down) as necessary to achieve a level of at least 1.2 mEq/L. In patients over 60 or those with possible renal impairment, the lower starting dose is indicated. Response in acutely manic states may require five to 14 days to occur even at an adequate blood level. As blood levels stabilize, their frequency may be decreased to two to three times a week initially and eventually to once a week as both blood levels and the clinical condition level out. If no clinical response occurs within four weeks, it is safe to assume that lithium will not be effective in the acute episode.

In practice, because lithium alone is not enough in excited manic patients, most acutely psychotic patients will be on antipsychotic drugs concurrently prior to lithium therapy or will have antipsychotics added if lithium does not have some obvious clinical effect in the first week. This combined therapy will, of course, confound the clinician's ability to judge whether or not lithium is having a significant clinical effect.

Other Current Target Symptoms

Here the situation is less urgent and an initial dosage of 300 mg two or three times a day seems adequate. There are some patients who end up benefitting from lithium who present with histories of marked lithium intolerance that appears to have been caused by overaggressive initial dosing. In these less urgent situations, a level of 0.5-0.8 mEq/L is probably adequate and less frequent blood levels are needed. It is also important to remember that one is treating a patient, not a blood level, and that both clinical status and side effects need frequent careful monitoring. Some patients report clear symptom relief at levels around 0.5 mEq/L; it seems senseless to push them to higher serum levels. Similarly, keeping a patient chronically nauseated, mentally dulled, and grossly tremulous just to maintain an "adequate" blood level is counterproductive in almost all situations.

In chronic disorders manifesting overt current target psychopathology—depression, schizophrenia, cyclothymic frequent mood shifts, irascibility with frequent temper outbursts—trials of about four weeks with adequate or highest tolerated blood levels are usually sufficient to determine whether or not lithium will be clinically useful.

Maintenance Therapy

In patients who are in remission and are being stabilized on lithium to avert future psychotic episodes, one can begin at even lower dosages (one or two 300 mg doses a day); weekly serum levels are often sufficient during dosage adjustment. Again, the goal is to find a well-tolerated blood level as close to 0.8 mEq/L as possible. It is still unclear whether better prophylaxis occurs at higher serum levels. This seems reasonable and, in one major NIMH collaborative study, patients maintained at 0.8 mEq/L and above had fewer recurrences than patients stabilized at lower levels.

However, many clinicians report satisfactory prophylaxis at lower levels in some patients. Once a patient on maintenance lithium is stabilized adequately on weekly serum levels for a few weeks, monthly levels are sufficient, and after six months to a year of stability, levels every two to three months may suffice.

Once a patient has a stable daily dose, this can be spread over the day in any suitable regimen. Usually twice a day—morning and bedtime—is convenient and well tolerated, and dosages are less likely to be forgotten or overlooked. It has been suggested, but not proven, that once a day dosage may be associated with less polyuria. Gastric irritation after each dose is the major reason for spreading medication into three or four smaller administrations a day. Such regimens are common (and logistically easy) in hospitalized patients who are sometimes discharged on these regimens through inadvertence when a simpler regimen would suffice and might be taken more reliably after the patient is discharged home.

Reinstitution of Lithium Therapy

In patients who have responded in the past to lithium but have stopped the drug for weeks or months, it is clinically reasonable to place them immediately back on their prior dosage without retitrating if there is no reason to believe kidney function has changed in the interim. Frequent blood level monitoring should be reinstituted.

Dose Prediction and Dose Requirements

Several papers have described techniques for predicting the optimal dosage of lithium from a loading dose followed by several level determinations over the next 24 hours. These techniques can be used but do not seem to us to be worth the extra effort required.

Specific Clinical Indications

Mania. There is no final, conclusive statement possible about the use of lithium as a sole or primary drug treatment of acute mania. Lithium alone is clearly more effective than placebo and probably as effective as an antipsychotic in less severely excited manic patients. It is probably less effective than an antipsychotic in very hyperactive, disturbed, psychotic manic, or schizoaffective patients. However, given the risk of tardive dyskinesia with antipsychotics, a few clinicians opt to use lithium alone or with other less conventional antimanic agents such as clonazepam, L-tryptophan, or carbamazepine to avoid antipsychotics. Others start all manic patients routinely on an antipsychotic on the assumption that this will produce the most rapid control of psychopathology or aid in patient management. Many clinicians will then add lithium, either on the first day of drug therapy or after the mania has begun to respond to antipsychotics to stabilize the patient on both drugs. When the patient is clearly much improved, some clinicians will gradually taper the antipsychotic so that the patient will be on lithium alone at the end of the episode. In patients whose hospitalizations are brief, both medications will be in use at discharge and the tapering of the antipsychotic will be done in the community.

In patients with several prior manic episodes, the past history of drug response may be a guide to treatment of the new episode. On the other hand, in a patient with only a single typical manic episode, one can justify using only an antipsychotic and later instituting lithium if further affective episodes occur.

The problem of severe neurotoxicity reported mainly with the combined use of haloperidol and lithium in psychotic excitement deserves comment here. It is usually characterized by gross tremor, confusion, delirium, and sometimes dyskinesia. It can occur with lithium in combination with other neuroleptics. Similar states can occur with lithium toxicity alone. However, this severe complication is very rare and is mainly a reason to observe patients in combination treatment carefully and to stop both drugs at once if severe neurotoxic signs begin to emerge. One suspects that haloperidol-lithium toxicity is relatively more common because haloperidol is widely used in the treatment of mania. Again there is no compelling evidence that haloperidol is more effective than other neuroleptics in mania, and the severe neurotoxicity has been observed on other antipsychotics combined with lithium. If clinicians are seriously concerned about the lithium-haloperidol toxicity, this combination can readily be avoided, but clinical experience suggests that the combination is worth trying if the clinician prefers haloperidol in mania.

Schizophrenia.   There is reasonable evidence that lithium, at serum levels in the 0.8-1.1 mEq/L range, is useful in combination with an antipsychotic in schizoaffective patients, some of whom are considered atypical bipolar patients. This poorly defined group of conditions includes patients with chronic symptoms of psychosis between episodes as well as patients with reasonably good interepisode adjustment who show florid non-affect-consonant delusions and hallucinations during excited episodes. In both cases, if overactivity, insomnia, pressured speech, irritability, or other common manic symptoms are present during the episode, lithium is a reasonable drug therapy to add to an antipsychotic. In the few controlled studies in which lithium is added to an antipsychotic in schizophrenic patients with or without manic symptoms, lithium is often more effective, on the average, than placebo.

In some chronically impaired schizophrenics without more than the usual amount of affective overlay, lithium will produce useful but limited additional improvement when added to an antipsychotic regimen. This happens often enough to make a trial of lithium easily justifiable in any treatment-resistant schizophrenic patient, although perhaps only one in five will show clinical improvement. There is also a subgroup of chronic schizophrenics with brief episodic angry outbursts in whom lithium appears to act by decreasing impulsive anger rather than by reducing the level of psychosis.

However, in chronic treatment-resistant psychotic patients, drug treatments are often added and continued for months or years even if no obvious clinical response or only a trivial improvement has occurred, in the hope that the extra drugs might be helping. There seems little justification for continuing such a use of lithium for longer than six months if no clinical benefit is apparent.

Recurrent Bipolar Disorder. There is excellent evidence that lithium carbonate is more effective than placebo in preventing the recurrence of affective episodes, either manic or depressive, in bipolar patients. However, only half or maybe fewer of such patients have complete suppression of all episodes even with excellent medication compliance. Further, at least some of the patients who have manic recurrences on maintenance lithium are blamed for noncompliance unjustifiably—the noncompliance is probably secondary to a recurrence of mania rather than vice versa. In addition, some patients respond to lithium with suppression of mania but with continuing episodes of depression; others show only a partial reduction in severity in both phases. We have seen several patients who had been on lithium for several years and did badly, continuing to have episodes of mania and depression; they were judged to be lithium nonresponders but were clearly even worse when lithium therapy was abandoned as ineffective. Rapid-cycling bipolar patients generally do less well on lithium than patients with less frequent or regular episodes, but even these patients can have the severity of their episodes modulated.

In initiating maintenance "prophylactic" lithium therapy, both patient and, where available, spouse or significant other need careful instruction about the purposes and requirements of lithium therapy and possible side effects and complications. There is some evidence that continuing involvement of bipolar patients and their spouses in couples groups or of single patients in lithium support groups is helpful in maintaining intelligent drug compliance and in helping patients handle past, current, and future problems.

Many bipolar patients, when contemplating maintenance lithium therapy, ask, "Will I have to take lithium forever?" There are two issues here. One is whether patients ever stop having recurrent manic and depressive episodes once several episodes have occurred, and the other is whether abruptly stopping lithium will trigger an affective episode which might not otherwise occur. The evidence from placebo substitution studies in patients already stabilized successfully on lithium maintenance is that relapses occur with considerable frequency with about half the patients relapsing within six months. Other, uncontrolled, studies have reported small series of patients who relapse floridly within a few days. We suspect the latter consequence is unusual but may be real in some patients and may account for some of the florid relapses seen in patients on maintenance lithium who experiment with stopping (or forget to take) their medication for a few days. In our experience, stopping lithium abruptly for two or three days in patients who have developed uncomfortable symptoms of lithium toxicity has never led to a florid relapse.

The whole area of lithium discontinuation is not well understood but most clinicians assume that essentially all bipolar patients who are stable on lithium need to continue the medication indefinitely. One wonders, however, whether a trial off lithium could be worth trying in patients who have really stabilized both their illnesses and their life circumstances for several years and in whom there is some evidence that prior episodes were precipitated by stresses which are no longer present. Such trials off lithium need to be discussed with the patient's family in detail. Given the occasional rapid relapses observed on sudden discontinuation, slowly tapering the drug by 300 mg a day each month may be indicated on grounds of general conservativism.

Depressive Disorders.   Some depressions improve on lithium alone (and some on placebo alone). Lithium alone has not been proven to be consistently effective in the treatment of depression, but some experts assert that lithium is particularly effective in depressions in bipolar patients. So few bipolar patients are seen these days in a depression and off lithium that this proposition is almost untestable. There are also recent studies suggesting that adding lithium to a tricyclic antidepressant or an MAOI in a patient who has not responded to the antidepressant after three to six weeks may lead to a clear, favorable response (see Chapters 3 and 9). There is also some suggestion that mixed affective states with dysphoria, agitation, insomnia, and pressured thoughts and speech may be helped by lithium. It is also worth trying in patients with rapid, unstable mood shifts occurring within a day (emotionally unstable character disorder) or in patients meeting *DSM-III* criteria for cyclothymic disorder.

In patients with bipolar disorder, the evidence is that combining imipramine with lithium in maintenance therapy may slightly increase the risk of manic relapse. In recurrent unipolar depression, the evidence from large-scale studies is mixed on the exact prophylactic potential of lithium; some showed lithium and imipramine to be equally effective, whereas the most recent study showed imipramine to be superior to lithium but both to be superior to placebo. The combination of imipramine and lithium was not superior to imipramine alone. Thus, clinicians may choose to use lithium alone to prevent recurrence of depression.

As a drug useful in episodic affective disorder, lithium has been tried in paramenstrual dysphoria with some success, but the vagueness of the condition and its alleged placebo responsivity make this potential indication a bit suspect.

Rage and Irritability. There is a reasonable clinical literature, mainly but not exclusively uncontrolled, which supports the proposition that some patients with episodic uncontrolled violent rage outbursts respond to lithium. The drug is certainly not always effective in such cases, but these predominantly nonpsychotic behavior disorders often present such appalling clinical problems that any drug with a chance of helping substantially deserves a trial. We concur with Tupin's general position that in violent prisoners and the like lithium controls outbursts of rage that are untriggered or triggered instantaneously by minor stimuli; however, lithium does not affect premeditated aggressive behavior. The drug is helpful in some patients with organic disorders or mental retardation who display episodic angry outbursts.

Alcoholism.   There are clinical claims that lithium is useful in episodic, binge drinkers in preventing their dipsomanic episodes. Certainly some patients presenting as alcoholics have underlying bipolar or unipolar recurrent affective disorders and drink to excess to anesthetize their depression or to slow their mania; such patients should benefit from lithium. Controlled studies by Merry and by Kline, although weak in their findings, suggest that some alcoholics with depressive symptoms do better on lithium than on placebo over time. However, most alcoholics show some dysphoria during detoxification, and many have the recall of their past psychiatric histories well muddled by alcoholism; these complications make clear differentiation of affective disorder difficult in chronic alcoholics.

On balance, it seems preferable to reserve lithium therapy for alcoholics with a documented history of recurrent bipolar disorder.

Side Effects

Neuromuscular and Central Nervous System Effects.   The most common side effect in lithium therapy is tremor, principally noticed in the fingers. It resembles intention, coffee-induced, or familial tremor in frequency, being faster than pseudoparkinsonian tremor. When tremor is severe enough to affect handwriting, the writing is usually jagged and irregular, but not micrographic as in parkinsonism. Tremor is sometimes worse at peak lithium blood level and can be ameliorated by dosage rearrangement. Dosage reduction can often be used to bring the blood level low enough to make tremor either absent or mild and inconspicuous. If there is good reason to maintain a serum lithium level which causes a disturbing degree of tremor, propranolol at doses from 30 to 160 mg a day can be used to reduce the tremor. Some patients on lithium also develop cog-wheeling and mild signs of parkinsonism, and naturally occurring parkinsonism can be aggravated. With toxic lithium levels, gross tremulousness and ataxia with dysarthria will occur, with the patient appearing grossly neurologically disordered and often confused or, less often, delirious at the same time. Seizures occur rarely with severe lithium toxicity.

Some patients on lithium complain of slowed mentation and forgetfulness and, on testing, a memory deficit has been found. Although such patients are often suspected or accused of "using" such symptoms to avoid necessary lithium therapy, our impression is that these complaints are often real and constitute a basis for lowering the dosage or trying another therapy. Some patients worry that they may become less creative on lithium. Schou, however, has asserted that maintenance lithium therapy does not generally affect artistic creativity.

With all of the above neurological symptoms, stopping lithium will lead to a disappearance of the side effects, but the symptoms and signs may persist for two to five days, longer than one would think it would take for the offending lithium to be cleared from the body.

Gastrointestinal Effects. Chronic nausea and watery diarrhea can occur together or separately as signs of lithium toxicity. Episodic nausea occurring only after each dose may be due to local gastric irritation and may be relieved by taking lithium with food. Shifting to a different lithium preparation may also be helpful.

Weight Gain and Endocrine Effects. Some patients gain weight progressively on lithium. The mechanisms are unclear. A few patients have overt edema and/or lose several pounds rapidly when lithium is stopped. In more patients, increased appetite with resulting weight gain is the problem, and attempting to control weight with dietary regulation is often very difficult for the patient. Why some patients will gain 40 to 60 pounds on lithium while others stay slim without any effort is totally bewildering.

Most patients show a transitory decrease in thyroid levels early in lithium therapy, and a very few show goiter with normal thyroid studies except for elevated thyroid-stimulating hormone levels. Some clinicians add thyroid supplements at this point. However, we recommend using thyroid primarily in patients with marked goiter or in those with associated anergy. Persistent hypothyroidism on lithium can occur but it is rare; it requires thyroid medication.

Renal Effects. Lithium causes polyuria with secondary polydipsia to a noticeable degree in some patients, roughly perhaps in one out of five. In a few patients this may extend to severe renal diabetes insipidus with urine volume up to eight liters a day and difficulty in concentrating urine and maintaining adequate lithium serum levels. This range of renal effects is due to a decrease in the resorption of fluid from the distal tubules of the kidney. It can be treated, obviously, by lowering the dose of lithium or stopping the drug. In most, but not all cases, the renal effect wears off in days or weeks after lithium is stopped.

An alternate strategy in patients in whom lithium is clearly necessary and the polyuria is distressing is to add a thiazide diuretic. Chlorthiazide at a dose of 500 mg a day is well documented to decrease lithium clearance by about 50 percent. Thus one can rationally add 500 mg of chlorthiazide a day and must then reduce the lithium dosage by 50 percent and then carefully restabilize the desired lithium level. This maneuver is sometimes effective, as it is in naturally occurring nephrogenic diabetes insipidus and can be used in milder but troublesome cases of polyuria. Amiloride (Midamor) has recently been reported to decrease lithium-induced polyuria without, allegedly, affecting either potassium excretion or lithium serum levels. If this is tried, it is still better to check lithium levels carefully while assessing amiloride's effectiveness in improving renal resorption of fluid and decreasing urine volume, because a few patients on the amiloride-lithium combination *do* get elevated lithium serum levels.

The prohibition in *PDR* against combining lithium with at least thiazide diuretics is much overstated. If a patient is stabilized on lithium at a clinically useful blood level (e.g., 0.8 mEq/L) and a thiazide diuretic is added in ignorance, the lithium level can double and the patient may suddenly develop signs of lithium toxicity. However, we see no problem in starting lithium therapy in a patient already stabilized on a thiazide diuretic; even patients on the artificial kidney have been successfully treated with lithium. Renal impairment before lithium therapy means the clinician should raise the dose very slowly and cautiously with careful serum level monitoring.

A different and potentially more serious renal problem is interstitial nephritis, first reported by Danish workers in 1977. It is characterized by renal scarring and glomerular destruction. Currently, the problem no longer seems as threatening or bothersome as it did initially. Major renal impairment manifested by seriously decreased creatinine clearance appears to be quite rare—we are aware only of a handful of such patients observed at McLean Hospital to have had any significant decrease in creatinine clearances since the phenomenon was first described. All but one of these had either serum creatinine levels or creatinine clearance which were only slightly abnormal. Reports from Europe and the United States tend to be confirmatory—no patients have been reported to have had life-threatening kidney dysfunction. Some patients with chronic affective disorders who have never been on lithium show renal pathology, and not all kidney dysfunction on lithium is necessarily caused by lithium.

Still, it is worth checking kidney function periodically in

patients on maintenance lithium. The "best" way would be to measure creatinine clearance periodically, but logistical problems and doubts about patient reliability in 24-hour urine collection have caused this procedure to be generally disfavored. Serum creatinine itself offers a reasonable indicator of kidney function since creatinine production is a function of muscle mass and is not affected by diet. Lithium serum level at constant intake is also a function of glomerular filtration. Watching both measures periodically should allow detection of early changes in glomerular function.

If the lithium dosage requirement gradually decreases and serum creatinine is persistently elevated, then a nephrology consultation is indicated. Even if renal impairment appears to exist, the decision whether to stop lithium therapy should be based on the total situation. Patients who have major benefit from maintenance lithium and either mild renal deficit or a kidney problem that may not be lithium related can be kept on lithium with more frequent monitoring of kidney function.

Drug Effects on Lithium Excretion.   In addition to the effect of thiazide diuretics (or low salt diets, including fasting completely) in decreasing lithium excretion, xanthine diuretics including caffeine probably *increase* lithium excretion. High coffee intake in hospitalized manic patients could account for the difficulty sometimes encountered in achieving therapeutic serum lithium levels even with very large lithium carbonate dosages (e.g., 2400 mg a day) in such patients.

Indomethacin and phenylbutazone have been reported to significantly decrease lithium excretion in humans; all the newer nonsteroidal antiinflammatory drugs should be viewed with suspicion. If a lithium-maintained patient requires such drug therapy, lithium levels should be closely monitored and the patient should be observed for possible increases in toxic symptoms.

We have seen one patient on lithium who received a course

of metronidazole therapy and has, ever since, shown a clear though clinically unimportant increase in serum creatinine into the abnormal range plus a decrease in the dose of lithium needed to maintain her old serum lithium levels. There is a similar case in the literature.

Cardiovascular Effects. Cases have been reported in which a "sick sinus node" syndrome has been brought on by lithium. This complication is very rare and probably not predictable unless the condition antedates lithium therapy. Baseline cardiograms are desirable in older patients or patients with any history at all of cardiac dysfunction.

Dermatologic Effects. A wide variety of diverse rashes have been described with lithium. Aggravation of preexisting or dormant psoriasis is well documented, and a dry noninflamed papular eruption is relatively common on maintenance lithium. Both zinc sulfate and tetracycline have been tried as treatments for this with variable success. Other less typical (for lithium) rashes of an itchy, presumably allergic nature can occur and often disappear if the specific lithium brand being used is changed; presumably these are allergic reactions to some ingredient in the capsule or tablet other than the lithium itself. Alopecia can occur in patients on lithium, but the hair often regrows either on or off lithium.

Other Side Effects. A variety of strange but rare symptoms can occur on lithium which sometimes turn out to be lithium related. At least they disappear when lithium is stopped and return when it is reinstituted, a reasonable though not infallible test of the drug-relatedness of any odd treatment-emergent symptom or sign on any drug.

Lithium in Pregnancy

Lithium is the only psychoactive nonanticonvulsant drug reliably associated with a specific birth defect, Ebstein's anomaly. This serious cardiac abnormality is not common (about 3 percent) in children born to mothers on lithium but is much more frequent in lithium babies than in the population at large. Other cardiac defects can also occur in lithium babies. This risk needs to be discussed with female patients on lithium who either are planning to get pregnant or are already pregnant (see Chapter 12).

Lithium Information

A lithium information center exists at the University of Wisconsin in Madison. Its telephone number is (608) 263–6171. The staff is most helpful in conducting focused literature searches for a small fee and can provide interested clinicians with helpful answers to a very wide variety of questions about lithium problems encountered in their practice.

ANTICONVULSANTS

In the past decade, increasing attention has been paid to the use of classic anticonvulsant medications to promote mood stabilization. The application of these agents stems from a number of observations on the psychiatric sequelae of temporal lobe epilepsy, including hallucinations, angry outbursts, religiosity, etc. These spurred on the application of phenytoin in the 1950s in psychiatric patients with, at best, equivocal results. In more recent years, several groups have further suggested that psychiatric symptoms could emanate from limbic seizures and that kindling phenomena could play a major role in the development of psychoses and psychiatric disorders. Understandably, then, a number of reports have emerged that other anticonvulsant agents (e.g., carbamazepine), which act more preferentially on temporal lobe or limbic systems, are effective in patients with manic-depressive illness, particularly in acute mania. Three compounds—carbamazepine, valproic acid, and clonazepam—have re-

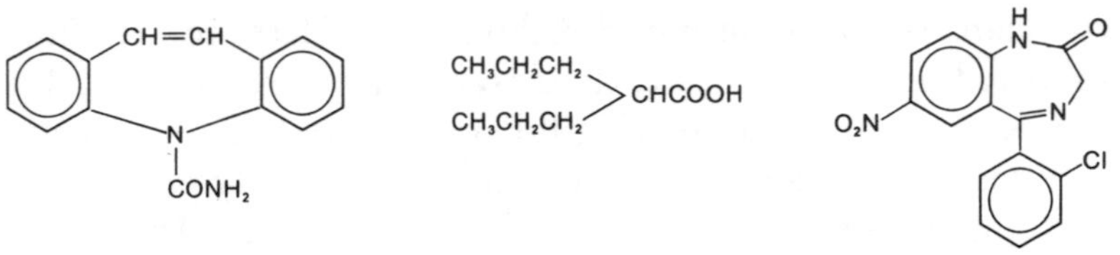

Carbamazepine   Valproic Acid   Clonazepam

Figure 5-1. Chemical Structures of Thymoleptic Anticonvulsants

ceived the lion's share of attention (Figure 5-1), although many of the available anticonvulsants may eventually prove useful in treating mood disorders. Of these, carbamazepine has been best studied as a long-term maintenance therapy.

Carbamazepine was originally synthesized in 1957 and introduced into the European market in the early 1960s as a treatment for epilepsy, particularly involving the temporal lobes. Subsequently, it became widely used as a treatment for "tic douloureux"—trigeminal neuralgia. Its use for manic-depressive illness stems from the early 1970s when Japanese researchers reported it was effective in many bipolar patients, including patients who were refractory to lithium. In 1980, Ballenger and Post reported that carbamazepine was effective in a double-blind crossover trial in acute bipolar patients. More recently, Kishimoto et al. (1983) reported that it was also effective in maintenance therapy.

Valproic acid, also introduced originally in Europe, was first inferred to be an active antiseizure medication in the early 1960s. In the 1970s, because of public outcry in the United States by parents of children with refractory epilepsy, the drug was approved by the FDA on a somewhat accelerated schedule. Its application to manic-depressive illness followed the reports on the use of carbamazepine in manic-depressive illness and was initially reported by Lambert et al. in 1975 and by Emrich et al. in 1984.

Clonazepam, a benzodiazepine that was originally introduced in the late 1970s as a treatment for myoclonic and akinetic seizures, has recently also been used by a number of clinicians to promote mood stabilization. Here, too, its use followed on the heels of carbamazepine and was initiated by physicians who were looking for potentially less toxic medications or for regimens that could be more easily prescribed in combination with other psychotropic agents. This is of particular practical importance since the other anticonvulsants often lower plasma levels of psychotropic drugs via induction of the liver enzymes.

Clinical Indications

The anticonvulsants are obviously indicated in the treatment of seizure disorders in children or adults. However, the three anticonvulsants we will concentrate on enjoy somewhat unique indications for specific types of seizure disorders. Carbamazepine is indicated for partial-complex seizures (e.g., temporal lobe epilepsy), generalized grand mal tonic-clonic seizures, and epileptic patients refractory to other agents. As indicated above, carbamazepine also enjoys an approved use for trigeminal neuralgia. Valproic acid is indicated for simple and complex absence seizures and as an adjunct in patients with multiple types of epilepsy. Clonazepam's indications include akinetic and myoclonic seizures, refractory absence seizures, and Lennox-Gastaut Syndrome (a variant of petit mal epilepsy).

The use of these agents as a mood stabilizer to prevent or treat episodes of mania or depression represents a non-FDA-approved, but potentially beneficial, "use" for all three drugs. In addition, carbamazepine has been proposed as a treatment for dysphoria, episodic violence or wrist cutting, borderline personality disorder, chronic pain, and diabetes insipidus. Moreover, carbamazepine may be useful as an adjunct to antipsychotic treatment in schizophrenic patients.

Names and Structures

Carbamazepine is manufactured and marketed in the United States under the trade name of Tegretol; valproic acid is marketed as Depakene or Depakote; and clonazepam is marketed as Klonopin. (Until recently, the brand name was Clonopin; however, the manufacturer changed the spelling to avoid confusion with Clonidine [see Chapter 6].) All three drugs are still under patent, so generic forms are not currently available. Structures are shown in Figure 5-1. Available formulations are summarized in Table 5-A.

Dosage Schedules

The dosage scheduling of the anticonvulsant medications for mood stabilization is still in some debate. For example, whereas higher dosages and serum levels have been advocated for carbamazepine's thymoleptic effect than for its antiseizure effect, many patients achieve mood stabilization when the drug is prescribed using lower antiseizure regimens. The antiseizure regimen calls for dosages beginning at 200 mg BID with gradual increases to a maximum of 1200-1600 mg/day in divided dosages. Therapeutic antiepileptic serum levels range between 4 and 8 mg/L. In contrast, Ballenger and Post (1980) point to dosages as high as 2000 mg/day to achieve what they believed was a therapeutic antimanic serum level of 8-12 mg/L. However, a number of earlier open-label studies reported that lower serum levels were frequently associated with thymoleptic benefit. In our experience, many patients respond at carbamazepine levels of 6-8 mg/L, and achieving levels >10 mg/L is often difficult.

We recommend beginning patients at 200 mg BID for two days and increasing to 200 mg TID for five days. At that point, a serum level should be obtained and dosage can be increased by 200 mg every four to seven days, depending on side effects, clinical response, and serum level obtained. Carbamazepine may induce liver enzymes after two to three weeks, resulting in a drop in blood level at constant dose and requiring further dosage adjustment.

Valproic acid has been less well studied with regard to its

mood-stabilizing properties. A reasonable regimen is to begin at 250 mg BID and to increase at a rate of 250 mg every four days up to the recommended antiseizure maximum of 60 mg/kg/day. In our experience, patients rarely require more than 1000-1500 mg/day. Here, too, drug serum levels can be used, but these are less meaningful than with carbamazepine.

Clonazepam has only recently been used for mood stabilization. The dosage range is 1.5-2.0 mg/day for control of seizures but even higher dosages (up to 40 mg/day) have reputedly been used for mood stabilization with other medications in acutely manic patients. The starting dosage in patients who are not acutely manic should begin at 0.5 mg BID-TID with increases of 0.5-1.0 mg every three days until stabilization occurs. Neurologists commonly find that the drug sedates their patients; in contrast, manic patients often appear to tolerate the drug better. However, patients vary widely in their ability to tolerate the drug, and we recommend that clinicians aim for dosages of 1.5-6 mg/day. Some 30 percent of myoclonic patients develop tolerance to the drug; similar studies have not been carried out in psychiatric patients. Obviously, as with any other drug that may induce tolerance, we recommend that clinicians adopt a conservative approach to prescribing and discontinuing the drug.

Our experience has been that these drugs can be most useful in two types of situations: 1) for acute mania and to prevent future manic episodes; and 2) for atypical depression—patients with depression who demonstrate depersonalization, perceptual distortions, history of seizures on or off psychotropic medications, and borderline personality features. For both situations, these drugs may prove of particular benefit in patients who fail to respond to more standard treatments—e.g., lithium carbonate, tricyclic antidepressants, etc.

Should these agents prove effective during a given episode, they should be prescribed for maintenance as one might a primary agent. Thus, in the manic or depressed patients who respond, the drug may be prescribed on a longer range basis to prevent early relapse as with other agents. However, the longer term use of these agents for mood stabilization has not been well studied. Thus, clinicians who use any of these agents for longer term maintenance should monitor their patients for any side effects. As with any maintenance schedule, lower dosages may prove effective, and it appears prudent for physicians to maintain patients on the lowest effective dose. When stopping the medication, tapering of the drug appears wise as with other thymoleptic agents, since rebound and withdrawal phenomena may occur.

Modes of Action

The modes of action of antiseizure drugs as thymoleptics are not clear, and considerable research continues as to their pharmacological actions in both neurologic and psychiatric disorders. Overall, antiseizure medications block the spread of seizure foci via inhibition of the firing of neurons by one of many possible mechanisms. If the purported theories that limbic firing, discharges, or kindling may produce various psychiatric symptoms is correct, blocking the aberrant firing of such structures and its spread would be of obvious importance. More specifically, pharmacologic properties of each of the three drugs highlighted in this chapter appear particularly intriguing for psychiatry. For one, carbamazepine, which has a tricyclic structure, is a potent blocker of norepinephrine reuptake. This effect could play a greater role in carbamazepine's purported antidepressant than in its antimanic properties. For valproic acid, pre- and postsynaptic gamma-aminobutyric acid (GABA) effects have been described. As do other benzodiazepines (see Chapter 6), clonazepam binds to the benzodiazepine receptors that are coupled to GABA receptors. Carbamazepine may act as a GABA agonist as well.

Side Effects

Carbamazepine can produce a variety of side effects, including sedation, nausea, vomiting, ataxia, dizziness, and drowsiness. Of these, we have found sedation and drowsiness to be the most common. They tend to be dose related and can be most easily managed by increasing dosages gradually by beginning with dosages as low as 100 mg per day and increasing at the rate of 100 mg every three days up to 400 mg per day. If the patient is accommodating to sedation at 400 mg per day, dosage can then be increased more rapidly (by 200 mg every three days). In addition, carbamazepine also produces a variety of anticholinergic effects associated with tricyclic antidepressants.

Of particular concern are the bone marrow suppressing effects of carbamazepine, which occur to a clinically worrisome extent in up to 3 percent of patients. These include leukopenia, anemia, thrombocytopenia, and pancytopenia. For this reason, checking blood counts weekly or biweekly for three months seems reasonable. For longer term treatment, monitoring should be done monthly but more frequently if problems arise or are suspected. If, on monitoring, the white blood cell count dips below 3500–4000 WBC/mm, the drug should be stopped immediately and consultation sought from a hematologist (Joffe et al. 1985). Serious agranulocytosis and aplastic anemia are quite rare.

Valproic acid is less sedating than carbamazepine and exerts little in the way of anticholinergic side effects. The most common side effects are those involving nausea, vomiting, and anorexia, which occur in 15-20 percent of patients. There has been concern regarding hepatotoxicity, and periodic liver function tests are recommended. Many neurologists concentrate more on possible increases in bilirubin than on minor increases in transaminases.

Clonazepam's side-effect profile is similar to those of other benzodiazepines. The clinician should titrate dosages to help patients who develop the primary side effects of sedation and lethargy. Generally, dosage reduction and gradual escalation results in reasonable toleration of these untoward effects. For description of other possible side effects, the reader is referred to Chapter 6.

Bibliography

Altesman R, Cole JO: Lithium therapy: a practical review, in Psychopharmacology Update. Edited by Cole JO. Lexington, Mass, Collamore Press, 1980, pp 3–18

Amdisen A: Lithium and drug interactions. Drugs 24:133–139, 1982

Ayd F: Carbamazepine for aggression, schizophrenia and nonnaffective syndromes. International Drug Therapy Newsletter 19:9–12, 1984

Baestrup P, Schou M: Lithium as a prophylactic agent against recurrent depressions and manic-depressive psychosis. Arch Gen Psychiatry 16:162–172, 1967

Baldessarini RJ, Lipinski JF: Lithium salts: 1970–1975. Ann Intern Med 83:527–533, 1975

Ballenger JC, Post RM: Carbamazepine (Tegretol) in manic-depressive illness: a new treatment. Am J Psychiatry 137:782–790, 1980

Beckmann H, Haas S: High dose diazepam in schizophrenia. Psychopharmacology 71:79–82, 1980

Biederman J, Lerner Y, Belmaker RH: Combination of lithium carbonate and haloperidol in schizoaffective disorder. Arch Gen Psychiatry 36:327–333, 1979

Blackwell B: Patient compliance with drug therapy. N Engl J Med 289:249–252, 1973

Cade JF: Lithium salts in treatment of psychotic excitement. Med J Aust 36:349–352, 1949

Cole J, Gardos G, Gelernter J, et al: Lithium carbonate in tardive dyskinesia and schizophrenia, in Tardive Dyskinesia and Affective Disorders. Edited by Gardos G, Casey D. Washington, DC, American Psychiatric Press, 1984, pp 50–73

Davenport Y, Ebert M, Adland M, et al: Couples group therapy as an adjunct to lithium maintenance of the manic patient. Am J Orthopsychiatry 47:495–502, 1977

Davis J: Overview: maintenance therapy in psychiatry, II: affective disorders. Am J Psychiatry 133:1–13, 1976

Deandrea D, Walker D, Mehlmauer M, et al: Dermatological reactions to lithium: a critical review of the literature. J Clin Psychopharmacol 2:199–204, 1982

Delva N, Letemendia F: Lithium treatment in schizophrenia and schizoaffective disorders. Br J Psychiatry 141:387–400, 1982

DePaulo JR Jr, Correa EI, Sapir DG: Renal glomerular function and long-term lithium therapy. Am J Psychiatry 138:324–327, 1981

Emrich H, Okuma T, Muller A (eds): Anticonvulsants in Affective Disorders. Excerpta Medica International Congress Series No 626. Amsterdam, Excerpta Medica, 1984

Evans RW, Gualtiere T: Carbamazepine: a neuropsychological and psychiatric profile. Clin Neuropharmacol 8:221–241, 1985

Groff P: Long term lithium treatment and the kidney. Can J Psychiatry 25:535–541, 1980

Himmelhoch JM, Forest J, Neil JF, et al: Thiazide-lithium synergy in refractory mood swings. Am J Psychiatry 134:149–152, 1977

Himmelhoch JM, Poust RI, Mallinger AG: Adjustment of lithium dose during lithium-chlorthiazide therapy. Clin Pharmacol Ther 22:225–227, 1977

Jefferson JW, Greist JH: Primer of Lithium Therapy. Baltimore, Williams and Wilkins, 1977

Jefferson JW, Greist JH, Ackerman DL, et al: Lithium Encyclopedia for Clinical Practice, 2nd ed. Washington, DC, American Psychiatric Press, 1986

Jefferson JW, Greist JH, Baudhuin M: Lithium: interactions with other drugs. J Clin Psychopharmacol 1:124–134, 1981

Jenner F: Lithium and the question of renal damage. Arch Gen Psychiatry 36:888–890, 1979

Jeste D, Wyatt R: Therapeutic strategies against tardive dyskinesia. Arch Gen Psychiatry 39:803–816, 1982

Joffe R, Post R, Roy-Byrne P, et al: Hemotological effects of carbamazepine in patients with affective illness. Am J Psychiatry 142:1196–1199, 1985

Kishimoto A, Ogura C, Hazama H, et al: Long-term prophylactic effects of carbamazepine in affective disorder. Br J Psychiatry 143:327–331, 1983

Klein DF, Gittelman R, Quitkin F, et al: Diagnosis and Treatment of Psychiatric Disorders: Adults and Children, 2nd ed. Baltimore, Williams and Wilkins, 1980

Klein E, Bental E, Lerer B, et al: Carbamazepine and haloperidol v placebo and haloperidol in excited psychoses. Arch Gen Psychiatry 41:165–170, 1984

Kline NS, Wren JC, Cooper TB, et al: Evaluation of lithium therapy in chronic and periodic alcoholism. Am J Med Sci 268:15–22, 1974

Kripke D, Robinson D: Ten years with a lithium group. McLean Hospital Journal 10:l-ll, 1985

Lambert P, Carraz G, Borselli S, et al: Dipropylacetamide in the treatment of manic-depressive psychosis. L'Encephale 1:25–31, 1975

Lingjaerde O: Benzodiazepines in the treatment of schizophrenia, in The Benzodiazepines: From Molecular Biology to Clinical Practice. Edited by Costa E. New York, Raven Press, 1983, pp 369–381

Luby E: Reserpine-like drugs—clinical efficacy, in Psychopharmacology: A Review of Progress, 1957–1967. Edited by Efron D. Washington, DC, US Government Printing Office, 1968, pp 1077–1082

Mendels J: Lithium in the treatment of depression. Am J Psychiatry 133:373–378, 1976

Merry J, Reynolds CM, Bailey J, et al: Prophylactic treatment of alcoholism by lithium carbonate. Lancet 2:481–482, 1976

Modell J, Lenox R, Weiner S: Inpatient clinical trial of lorazepam for the management of manic agitation. J Clin Psychopharmacol 5:109–113, 1985

Ortiz A, Dabbagh M, Gershon G: Lithium: clinical use, toxicology and mode of action, in Clinical Psychopharmacology, 2nd ed. Edited by Bernstein J. Littleton, Mass, Wright PSG, 1984, pp 111–144

Post R: Carbamazepine's acute and prophylactic effects in manic and depressive illness: an update. International Drug Therapy Newsletter 17:5–10, 1982

Post RM, Uhde TW: Carbamazepine in bipolar illness. Psychopharmacol Bull 21:10–17, 1985

Prien R: Long-term prophylactic pharmacologic treatment of bipolar illness, in Psychiatry Update, vol 2. Edited by Grinspoon L. Washington, DC, American Psychiatric Press, 1983, pp 303–318

Prien R, Caffey E, Klett C: A comparison of lithium carbonate and chlorpromazine in the treatment of excited schizoaffectives. Arch Gen Psychiatry 27:182–189, 1972

Prien R, Caffey E, Klett C: A comparison of lithium carbonate and chlorpromazine in the treatment of mania. Arch Gen Psychiatry 26:146–153, 1972

Prien RF, Caffey EM Jr: Long-term maintenance drug therapy in recurrent affective illness: current status and issues. Diseases of the Nervour System 38:981–992, 1977

Prien R, Kupfer D, Mansky P, et al: Drug therapy in the prevention of recurrences in unipolar and bipolar affective disorders. Arch Gen Psychiatry 41:1096–1104, 1984

Quitkin F, Rifkin A, Klein DF, et al: Prophylaxis in unipolar affective disorder. Am J Psychiatry 133:1091–1092, 1976

Ramsey TA, Cox M: Lithium and the kidney. Am J Psychiatry 139:443–449, 1982

Rifkin A, Quitkin F, Carrillo C, et al: Lithium carbonate in emotionally unstable character disorder. Arch Gen Psychiatry 28:519–523, 1972

Robertson M, Trimble M: Major tranquilizers used as antidepressants—a review. J Affect Disord 4:173–193, 1982

Salzman C: The use of ECT in the treatment of schizophrenia. Am J Psychiatry 137:1032–1041, 1980

Schou M: The range of clinical uses of lithium, in Lithium in Medical Practice. Edited by Johnson FN, Johnson S. Baltimore, University Park Press, 1978

Schou M: Artistic productivity and lithium prophylaxis in manic-depressive illness. Br J Psychiatry 135:97–103, 1979

Sheard JH, Marini JL, Bridges CI, et al: The effect of lithium on impulsive aggressive behavior in man. Am J Psychiatry 133:1409–1413, 1976

Tilkian AG, Schroder JS, Kao JJ, et al: The cardiovascular effects of lithium in man. Am J Med 61:665–670, 1976

Tupin J: Management of violent patients, in Manual of Psychiatric Therapeutics. Edited by Shader R. Boston, Little, Brown, 1975, pp 125–133

Uhde T, Post R, Ballenger J, et al: Carbamazepine in the treatment of neuropsychiatric disorders, in Anticonvulsants in Affective Disorders. Edited by Emrich H, Okuma T, Muller A. Excerpta Medica International Congress Series No 626. Amsterdam, Excerpta Medica, 1984, pp 111–131

Vendsborg PB, Bech P, Rafaelson OJ: Lithium treatment and weight gain. Acta Psychiatr Scand 53:139–147, 1976

Yorkston N, Zaki S, Harvard C: Some practical aspects of using propranolol in the treatment of schizophrenia, in Propranolol and Schizophrenia. Edited by Roberts E, Amacher P. New York, Liss, 1978, pp 83–97

Antianxiety Agents

6

Anxiolytic agents are the most commonly used psychotropic drugs. The vast majority of prescriptions for these medications are issued by internists, family practitioners, and obstetricians. Psychiatrists write less than 20 percent of the prescriptions for anxiolytics in this country, reflecting, in part, the fact that the vast majority of anxious patients never see psychiatrists. Moreover, anxiolytics are prescribed for many varieties of patients who do not suffer from a primary anxiety disorder. Rather, they are prescribed for patients who present to primary care physicians with somatic complaints or true somatic disease.

Antianxiety agents may be divided into many subclasses, of which the benzodiazepines are the most frequently prescribed. Several of the subclasses of anxiolytics (e.g., benzodiazepines) include agents that are marketed primarily as hypnotics (e.g., flurazepam). The differentiation between anxiolytic and hypnotic drugs is somewhat artifactual, with many of the traditional anxiolytic agents (e.g., diazepam) enjoying sedative properties. In this guide we have separated the pharmacologic treatments of anxiety from those of insomnia—albeit somewhat artificially—since almost any sedative or antianxiety drug can be used at a low dose in the daytime for anxiety and at a high dose for difficulty in sleeping.

The first major anxiolytic group, the barbiturates, were developed as sedative/hypnotic and antiepileptic agents and were first introduced in the early 1900s. These drugs are also discussed extensively in the chapter on hypnotics (Chapter 7). Meprobamate was introduced almost 60 years later as a sedative/anxiolytic agent. Although these two classes have waned in use in recent years, they are still more commonly prescribed than one might imagine; meprobamate and phenobarbital represent approximately 7 percent of the anxiolytic market. Benzodiazepines, introduced in the early 1960s, dramatically changed the pharmacologic approach to anxiety. First developed as muscle relaxants, their anxiolytic/hypnotic properties and wider safety margin in overdosage and addictive potential quickly became apparent. These drugs now account for over 80 percent of the anxiolytic market. Less widely used pharmacologic approaches to anxiety include antihistamines and autonomic agents (e.g., beta blockers). The former act primarily via a general sedative action; the latter—which are becoming increasingly used—act by blocking peripheral or central noradrenergic activity and many of the manifestations of anxiety (tremor, palpitations, sweating, etc.). Several of the phenothiazines also have indications in anxiety, although here they have become less widely used in recent years for this purpose. Several antidepressants appear effective in both generalized anxiety disorder and panic disorder, and clomipramine, currently not available on the United States market, has been reported to be very effective in some patients with obsessive-compulsive disorder.

Benzodiazepines

Indications

In addition to anxiety, benzodiazepines are indicated for muscle relaxation, insomnia, status epilepticus (diazepam), myoclonic epilepsy (clonazepam), preoperative anesthesia, and alcohol withdrawal. One new member—the triazolo-benzodiazepine alprazolam—is also indicated for anxiety associated with depression (as is lorazepam), and recent studies have indicated alprazolam may also parallel imipramine and phenelzine in having both antipanic and antidepressant properties (see also Chapter 3).

Mode of Action

In recent years, considerable attention has been paid to the potential mode of action of benzodiazepines, spurred on by the identification of specific receptor sites. These sites, found in various brain regions, are coupled to GABA receptors. This receptor complex appears to mediate the anxiolytic, sedative, and anticonvulsant actions of the benzodiazepines. The location of specific receptors may be related to the relative anticonvulsant, anxiolytic, or sedative properties of the various benzodiazepines. Some pharmacologists have hypothesized that it may be possible to develop new compounds that bind more specifically to certain receptors and produce anxiolysis without sedation.

The triazolo-benzodiazepine alprazolam also appears to have effects on noradrenergic systems, causing down-regulation of postsynaptic beta receptors in reserpine-treated mice and increasing the activity of the N-protein in humans (the protein that couples the postsynaptic receptor to the intraneuronal energy system). These effects may help to explain the drug's antipanic and moderate antidepressant effects.

Subclasses

The anxiolytic benzodiazepines are commonly divided into three subclasses on the basis of structure: 2-keto (chlordiazepoxide, diazepam, prazepam, clorazepate, halazepam, and the hypnotic flurazepam); 3-hydroxy (oxazepam, lorazepam, and the hypnotic temazepam); and triazolo (alprazolam and

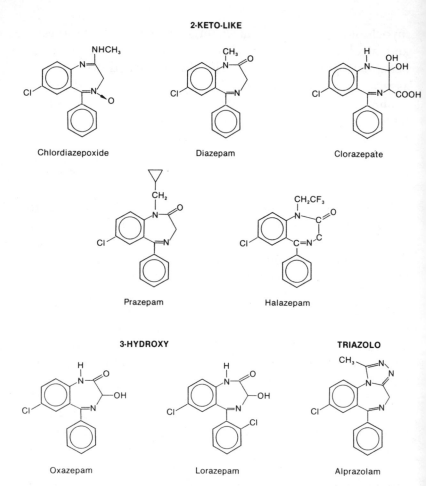

Figure 6-1. Chemical Structures of Anxiolytic Benzodiazepines

the hypnotic triazolam) (see Figure 6-1 and Table 6-A). The pharmacokinetic properties (i.e., half-lives) vary among these classes, in part reflecting differences in their modes of drug metabolism, as summarized in Table 6-B. The 2-keto drugs and their active metabolites are oxidized in the liver and, since this process is relatively slow, these compounds have relatively long half-lives. For example, the half-life of diazepam is approximately 40 hours. One active metabolite (desmethyldiazepam) has an even longer half-life: about 60 hours. Moreover, since desmethyldiazepam is further metabolized to oxazepam, which is also active as an anxiolytic (Table 6-A), diazepam imparts rather long-range sedative and anxiolytic effects.

Another interesting aspect of this class is that many of the marketed 2-keto drugs are prodrugs—they are themselves inactive but eventually form active metabolites. Thus prazepam, clorazepate, and halazepam are mere precursors for desmethyldiazepam—as is diazepam. Differences among these specific 2-keto compounds revolve around the rates of absorption and the specific active metabolites formed.

In contrast, the 3-hydroxy compounds are metabolized via direct conjugation with a glucoronide radical, a process that is more rapid than is oxidation and one which does not involve the formation of active metabolites. The two major examples of this subclass are oxazepam and lorazepam, which have considerably shorter half-lives (9 and 14 hours, respectively) than do their 2-keto counterparts. Similarly, the hypnotic temazepam has a half-life (eight hours) that is much shorter than flurazepam's.

The triazolo compounds are also oxidized; however, they appear to have more limited active metabolites and thus relatively shorter half-lives. The half-life of alprazolam is about 14 hours; that of the hypnotic triazolam is three to four hours.

The pharmacokinetic properties of benzodiazepines that are oxidized in the liver may be affected by other medications. Of particular note, cimetidine (Tagamet) and birth control pills inhibit liver oxidative enzymes and thus slow the degradation of the 2-keto and triazolo compounds. Clinicians should keep this in mind in treating anxious patients who are also taking these nonpsychotropic drugs.

Other differences among benzodiazepines revolve around their rates of absorption and distribution. For example,

Table 6-A. Benzodiazepines: Specific Compounds, Available Preparations, and Anxiolytic Dosage Ranges

Generic Name	Brand Name	Dosage Forms	Dosage Ranges (mg/day)*
2-Keto-			
chlordiazepoxide	Librium	Capsules: 5/10/25 mg	15–40
		Ampules: 20 mg/ml (5 ml)	50–100 once (25–50 TID)
	Libritabs	Tablets: 5/10/25 mg	15–40
clorazepate	Tranxene	Tablets: 3.75/7.5/15 mg	15–60
		Capsules: 3.75/7.5/15 mg	
	Tranxene SD	Tablets: 11.25/22.5 mg	11.25–45
diazepam	Valium	Tablets: 2/5/10 mg	5–40
		Parenteral: 5 mg/ml	
		(2 ml syringes)	
		(2 ml ampules)	
		(10 ml vials)	
	Valrelease	Capsules: 15 mg	15–30
		(slow release)	
halazepam	Paxipam	Tablets: 20/40 mg	60–160
prazepam	Centrax	Capsules: 5/10/20 mg	20–60
3-Hydroxy-			
lorazepam	Ativan	Tablets: 0.5/1/2 mg	1–6
		Parenteral: 2/4 mg/ml	1–2
		(1 and 10 ml vials)	
oxazepam	Serax	Tablets: 15 mg	45–120
		Capsules: 10/15/30 mg	
Triazolo-			
alprazolam	Xanax	Tablets: 0.25/0.5/1 mg	1–4

* Approximate dosage ranges. Some patients will require higher dosages; others may respond to dosages below the range.

Table 6-B. Benzodiazepines: Absorption and Pharmacokinetics

Generic Name	Oral Absorption	Major Active Components	Approximate Half-Life (hours)*
2-Keto-			
chlordiazepoxide	intermediate	chlordiazepoxide	20
		desmethylchlordiazepoxide	30
		demoxepam	Unknown
		desmethyldiazepam	60
clorazepate	fast	desmethyldiazepam	60
diazepam	fast	diazepam	40
		desmethyldiazepam	60
halazepam	slow	desmethyldiazepam	60
prazepam	slow	desmethyldiazepam	60
3-Hydroxy-			
lorazepam	intermediate	lorazepam	14
oxazepam	slow to intermediate	oxazepam	9
Triazolo-			
alprazolam	intermediate	alprazolam	14

* Based on ranges of half-lives reported in healthy young normal volunteers.

although prazepam and clorazepate are similar in structure and both are prodrugs of desmethyldiazepam, the two differ in terms of the metabolic processes required for absorption and thus in the rates at which they appear in blood (Table 6-B). Clorazepate and diazepam are rapidly absorbed and produce peaks in plasma levels more quickly than does prazepam, whose absorption is mediated via slower processes. Halazepam's conversion to desmethyldiazepam is also relatively slow.

The lipophilic and hydrophilic properties of these drugs also vary, resulting in pronounced differences in how quickly they work and for how long. Drugs that are more lipophilic (e.g., diazepam) will enter the brain more quickly—"turning on" the effect promptly, but "turning off" more quickly as well—as they disappear into body fat. Less lipophilic compounds (e.g., lorazepam) will produce clinical effects more slowly but may provide more sustained relief. These properties are largely independent of pharmacokinetics. Some drugs with long half-lives (e.g., diazepam) can also be highly lipophilic, providing rapid relief but for shorter periods than one might predict from half-life data alone. In contrast, lorazepam, which has a shorter half-life, is less lipophilic and turns on and off more slowly, potentially providing more sustained effects. In short, traditional half-life pharmacokinetics can be misleading and only tell a part of the story of how drugs work. In addition, investigators have begun to pay more attention to relative receptor affinity, a property that may play a more important role in determining the duration of action than previously thought. High-potency benzodiazepines, such as lorazepam and alprazolam, may have such high affinity that withdrawal symptoms may be far more intense than one might expect from inspecting other variables such as half-lives. Interestingly, oxazepam, which is similar in lipid solubility and half-life to lorazepam, appears to produce less in the way of withdrawal symptoms. This position has been most eloquently stated by Lader in the United Kingdom.

Although several of the benzodiazepines are available for parenteral usage (see Table 6-A), there is wide variability in the absorption properties of these compounds when given intramuscularly. For example, lorazepam is relatively rapidly absorbed when given intramuscularly. In contrast, chlordiazepoxide and diazepam are slowly absorbed. Lorazepam has become increasingly popular as an adjunctive treatment for agitation in acutely psychotic patients. Oral concentrate forms of benzodiazepines are not available in the United States.

Dosage Ranges

The efficacy of benzodiazepines in patients with symptomatic anxiety or diagnosable anxiety disorders has been established in double-blind, random assignment comparisons with placebo. When treating a patient with generalized anxiety disorder, the clinician should begin at approximately 2 mg TID of diazepam with increases as needed to a maximum regular daily dose of diazepam of 40 mg. A modal dose of diazepam for generalized anxiety disorder is 15-20 mg/day. Chlordiazepoxide has a much wider dosage range. Recommended starting dose is 5-10 mg po TID with a maximum of 60 mg/day for anxiety. The dosage of chlordiazepoxide used for acute alcohol withdrawal is much higher—50-200 mg/day. Generally, clinicians prescribe 25 mg every one to two hours until symptomatic relief or sedation occurs, up to a maximum of 200 mg/day. Dosage ranges of the anxiolytic benzodiazepines are listed in Table 6-A.

The use of alprazolam in panic patients may require higher dosages than those used in generalized anxiety disorder. Currently, alprazolam is approved in dosages up to 4 mg/day; however, some studies on panic disorder or depression have used doses of up to 10 mg/day. In our studies on depression, we have used the much higher dosage regimen, but we have been impressed that patients generally do not require more than 4-6 mg/day to respond and some are oversedated at 2-3 mg/day. Starting dosage of alprazolam in both generalized anxiety disorder and panic disorder should be 1.5 mg/day or less, given in divided doses with a gradual increase in dosage as tolerated by the patient. Although alprazolam may be unique in antipanic effects, other benzodiazepines have not been as well studied. One recent report indicated that 30 mg/day of diazepam was effective in ameliorating panic symptoms.

In patients who have occasional bouts of moderate anxiety ocurring only every few days or weeks, benzodiazepines are best used as prn medication. Diazepam's ability to act rapidly without prolonged sedation makes it particularly useful in such situations in patients not prone to drug abuse. Other benzodiazepines can also be used in this manner, of course.

One major area of debate revolves around how long to use these drugs for patients with significant anxiety. For those patients whose anxiety is more acute and is related to specific stressors, use of these agents should be directed at reduction of acute symptoms and thus prolonged use beyond one to two weeks is generally not required. However, patients with generalized anxiety disorder require longer treatment. We recommend treatment for three to four weeks at doses that provide relief, then reduction of dosage to the minimum needed for maintenance for the next one to two months, and then discontinuation when possible. Unfortunately, there are many patients who obtain relief from these drugs but who relapse when they are stopped. Yet, since there are patients who seem to do well on reasonable dosages over longer periods, the clinician may be faced with a difficult decision of how long to maintain the benzodiazepine. This dilemma is intensified by the observations that tolerance can develop to benzodiazepines, suggesting to some that the apparent relief experienced by patients reflects a nonspecific psychological effect.

Although tolerance is a real phenomenon, it is our belief that some patients actually do not develop tolerance but are still responding. We base this observation on the numbers of patients we have seen over the years who have functioned well on a given daily dose of benzodiazepine and have not found themselves escalating their total daily intake. In addition, it is our impression that animal and human models of tolerance may not be totally applicable to chronic anxiety per se; rather, they emphasize reinforcing self-administration of drug or ataxia produced in "normal" specimens but do not take into full account the biological and clinical status of the anxious patient. If possible, the clinician should attempt to taper the patient off benzodiazepines, using psychotherapy or behavior therapy to help patients deal with their anxiety. Some patients, however, may require continued pharmacologic intervention.

True longer term harmful effects of benzodiazepines have not been convincingly described. For example, Lader (1982) reported computed tomographic scan abnormalities in a series of patients who had taken benzodiazepines on a long-term basis. Although these observations could be interpreted as indicating that these drugs produce organic/structural changes in brain tissue (as chronic alcohol use does), an equally acceptable explanation is that some anxious patients who require chronic treatment with benzodiazepines may have neuropsychiatric disorders as evidenced by computed tomographic scan abnormalities. A recent study by Lucki et al. (in press) of patients on chronic long-term benzodiazepine treatment failed to show significant cognitive impairment on psychometric tests.

Are these drugs addictive? Do they produce withdrawal symptoms? Studies in animals indicate that benzodiazepines can reinforce use and can produce physical dependence and tolerance. However, they appear to be much less addictive than many other drugs—e.g., narcotics, barbiturates, alcohol, etc. Although a great deal of attention has been focused on the addictive properties and misuse of these drugs (particularly by nonphysicians), this is—paradoxically—less of an issue for psychiatrists treating anxiety disorder patients. Rather, it is of importance in addiction-prone individuals who often do not meet criteria for anxiety disorders.

Should one withdraw patients who have taken benzodiazepines regularly over longer periods? As a rule, this is sensible, reducing at a maximum rate of approximately 10 percent per day. (For alprazolam, reduction at a slower rate of 0.5 mg every three days may be required.) In their classic study of benzodiazepine withdrawal, Rickels et al. (1983) noted that patients who had been on benzodiazepines for more than eight months more frequently (43 percent) demonstrated withdrawal symptoms on abrupt discontinuation under double-blind conditions than did patients (5 percent) who were taking benzodiazepines for shorter periods.

Common withdrawal symptoms include jitteriness, anxiety, palpitations, clamminess, sweating, nausea, confusion, and heightened sensitivity to light and sound. Seizures represent the most worrisome of withdrawal reactions but fortunately are rare. No patients in the study by Rickels et al. experienced seizures. Seizures with abrupt diazepam withdrawal occur some five to seven days after stopping the drug and not within 24 hours, reflecting the long half-lives of diazepam and desmethyldiazepam. With shorter acting drugs (e.g., lorazepam and alprazolam), withdrawal symptoms emerge more rapidly—within two to three days. Thus with diazepam, physicians cannot be confident that seizures will not occur unless the patient has been off the drug at least one week. Any signs of withdrawal (even at day five) should be reviewed carefully, and consideration should be given to reinstituting the drug and then withdrawing it more gradually.

Side Effects

Compared with many other classes of psychotropic agents, benzodiazepines enjoy relatively favorable side effect profiles. The most common side effect is sedation, which is in part dose related and can be managed by reducing dosage. Other effects include dizziness, weakness, ataxia, anterograde amnesia, decreased motoric performance (e.g., driving), nausea, and slight hypotension. Fortunately, these drugs have a relatively wide safety margin, and deaths due to benzodiazepine ingestion alone are relatively rare. Most deaths that have involved these drugs have also been associated with ingestion of other agents—e.g., alcohol, tricyclic antidepressants, etc.

BARBITURATES

Thirty to forty years ago, the only medications widely used in psychiatric patients for the treatment of anxiety or agitation were in fact barbiturates. Longer acting barbiturates, such as phenobarbital or barbital, were widely used for daytime sedation, and shorter acting barbiturates with, presumably, more rapid onset of action, such as secobarbital, amobarbital, or pentobarbital, were widely used as hypnotics. (For further discussion of hypnotics, see Chapter 7.) Amobarbital (Figure 6-2) in particular was also widely used as a daytime sedative and, in combination with *d*-amphetamine, as a widely used mixed sedative and stimulant called Dexamyl, no longer available in the United States. In general clinical use at the present time, phenobarbital is the only barbituate that is widely used, and it is used essentially only in the treatment of epilepsy (see Figure 6-2). It has some efficacy as a daytime sedative and possibly as an antianxiety agent in doses of 15-30 mg three or four times a day and is also used as a long-acting sedative (the methadone of the barbiturate group) in some detoxification programs, withdrawing patients from shorter acting sedatives or occasionally from alcohol. In double-blind controlled clinical trials comparing phenobarbital with placebo and a benzodiazepine or meprobamate, phenobarbital generally came out slightly more effective than placebo and inferior to the newer antianxiety agents. In many

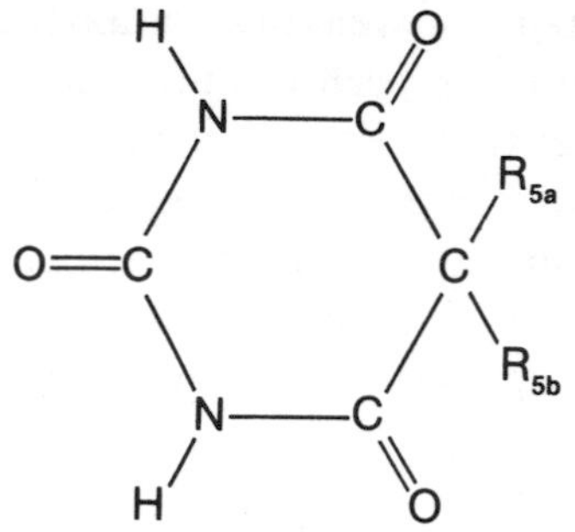

Compound	R_{5a}	R_{5b}
Amobarbital	ethyl	isopentyl
Aprobarbital	allyl	isopropyl
Butabarbital	ethyl	sec-butyl
Pentobarbital	ethyl	l-methylbutyl
Phenobarbital	ethyl	phenyl
Secobarbital	allyl	l-methylbutyl

Figure 6-2. General Chemical Formulas of the Barbiturates

such studies the dose of phenobarbital used was fixed and low, and its efficacy may well have been played down by the conditions of the trial. However, many patients find the sedative effect of phenobarbital rather dysphoric and unpleasant, and its utility as an antianxiety drug is therefore limited. In patients taking phenobarbital for epilepsy and more strikingly in children or even adults with a history of attentional deficit disorder, phenobarbital can in fact aggravate hyperactivity and disorganized behavior. Occasionally, increased hyperactivity and disturbed behavior in some children and adolescents can be traced to their taking antiasthmatics that contain phenobarbital.

On the other hand, it is quite possible that amobarbital or other relatively shorter acting barbiturates might be as effective as benzodiazepines in the daytime treatment of anxiety. Several enjoy indications for daytime sedation, and of these butabarbital (Butisol) is occasionally used in such a way. (See Table 6-C for preparations and Figure 6-2 for structures of the barbiturates.) No good controlled clinical trials have been done comparing such shorter acting and possibly less dysphoric and more euphoric barbiturates with benzodiazepines. There is, however, little point in carrying out such trials, since it is reasonably clear that the addiction and abuse liability of barbiturates is substantially greater than that of most benzodiazepines, even including diazepam. The barbiturates like amobarbital also have the disadvantage of the lethal dose being relatively low, perhaps 1000 mg taken in a single overdose, and the barbiturates induce enzymes which metabolize some other important medications. It is also possible but not proven that tolerance develops somewhat more rapidly to the barbiturates when taken in escalating dosages. In a classic study by Isbell et al. (1950), performed at the Addiction Research Center in Lexington in the 1940s, patients on very large daily doses of barbiturates managed to complain of going into withdrawal while being so ataxic and malcoordinated that they were falling down when they tried to walk and were slurring their speech. This suggests that the tolerance to the antianxiety and/or euphoriant effects of the barbiturates develops more rapidly than does tolerance to the drugs' effects on psychomotor functions. Very large doses of benzodiazepines taken chronically do not appear to have this property.

Sodium amobarbital (Amytal) as a parenteral solution is still of some value in psychiatry. When given intramuscularly to quiet agitated behavior in disturbed or psychotic patients, a dose of 100 mg is common with a range between 50 mg and 250 mg, based on the weight of the patient and the degree of excitement. It has one major advantage over parenteral antipsychotics such as chlorpromazine, haloperidol, or loxapine in that it acts more rapidly, perhaps in 10-

Table 6-C. Other Antianxiety/Daytime Sedative Agents*

Generic Name	Brand Name	Dosage Forms	Dosage Range (mg/day)
Barbiturates			
amobarbital	Amytal	Tablets: 15/30/50/100 mg Capsules: 65/200 mg Concentrate: 44 mg/5 ml (16 oz bottles) Parenteral: 250/500 mg vials	60–150 100
butabarbital	Buticaps Butisol	Capsules: 15/30 mg Tablets: 15/30/100/150 mg Concentrate: 30 mg/5 ml (16 oz bottles)	45–120
mephobarbital pentobarbital	Mebaral Nembutal	Tablets: 32/50/100/200 mg Capsules: 30/50/100 mg Concentrate: 20 mg/ml (16 oz bottles) Parenteral: 50 mg/ml (2 ml ampules, 20/50 ml vials)	150–200 90–120 150–200 once (up to 500)
phenobarbital	Multiple Generic	Tablets and Capsules: (multiple strengths)	30–120

			mg/day
Carbamates			
meprobamate	Equanil Miltown	Tablets: 200/400 mg Tablets: 200/400/600 mg Concentrate: 16 mg/ml drops, 20 mg/5 ml elixir Parenteral: multiple strength syringes, ampules, and vials	1200–1600
Noradrenergic Agents			
clonidine	Catapres	Tablets: 0.1/0.2/0.3 mg Parenteral: 1 mg/ml (1 ml ampules)	0.2–0.6
propranolol	Inderal	Tablets: 10/20/40/60/80/90 mg	60–160
Antihistamines			
hydroxyzine HCl	Atarax	Tablets: 10/25/50/100 mg Concentrate: 10 mg/5 ml (16 oz bottles)	200–400
hydroxyzine pamoate	Vistaril	Tablets: 25/50/100 mg Concentrate: 25 mg/5 ml Parenteral: multiple strength syringes and vials	200–400
			50–100

* For information regarding antidepressants as anxiolytics, see Chapter 3.

20 minutes and, when it acts, it tends to produce sleep rather than tranquilization. We know of no systematic study of the relative utility of amobarbital compared to either haloperidol or chlorpromazine in the treatment of acutely disturbed behavior requiring only a single injection. The advantage of amobarbital as noted is that it produces sleep relatively rapidly. The disadvantage is that when the patient awakens, there is no residual antipsychotic activity to modulate the patient's subsequent behavior. Although in the past amobarbital was administered intramuscularly several times a day through prolonged psychotic excitements, there is no real reason to believe that it is in fact regularly antipsychotic or has any prolonged benefit. There is some suggestion that too frequent use could result in either tolerance or, occasionally, delirium. It is quite possible that lorazepam, given intramuscularly in 1-2 mg doses, will prove as useful as, and safer than, amobarbital.

Intravenous amobarbital has been used in extreme emergency conditions in psychiatry to produce anesthetic-type sleep within a few minutes. A dose of 150-200 mg given over a period of three to five minutes intravenously could be used, and additional doses up to 500 mg could be given if 250 mg is not adequate to produce quiet sleep. If such "anesthetic" use of amobarbital is being prescribed, the physician should carefully watch the patient's breathing and vital signs and give the medication slowly to make sure that respiration is not suppressed. The major danger in addition to suppression of the respiratory center in such treatment is the occasional production of laryngospasm in patients with irritation of the larynx and upper respiratory system. Barbiturates can of course also produce crises in patients with acute intermittent porphyria.

Intravenous amobarbital in doses of 100-300 mg, sometimes higher, has been used also in psychiatric conditions to conduct Amytal interviews. When the amobarbital is injected slowly over five to 10 minutes in ordinary psychiatric patients, a state of relaxation and mild intoxication with slurred speech can be achieved during which patients will often talk more easily and more volubly about their problems and past experiences. Sometimes patients under these conditions will reveal material not previously told the psychiatrist. Although amobarbital has been called "truth serum," it is by no means certain that stories told by patients under the influence of amobarbital are likely to be any more truthful than stories told in the fully conscious state.

The Amytal interview was developed during World War II by Grinker and Spiegel (1945) as a treatment for severe combat fatigue. In the typical situation, soldiers emerged from combat essentially mute, shaking, paralyzed with fear, and looking blocked, dysphoric, and peculiar. They were either mute or unable to answer questions in more than monosyllables and appeared unable to cope emotionally with the traumatic events they had recently experienced. Under intravenous amobarbital, such soldiers often were able to give vivid and emotionally charged accounts of their horrifying experiences, and this form of catharsis often served to discharge their inner tensions and to enable them to function thereafter in a more normal and organized fashion with a substantially reduced level of anxiety. It is reasonable to believe that amobarbital might be of use in similar conditions which resemble some kind of acute traumatic stress syndrome encountered in clinical practice. Amytal interviews have also been used, often with some success, in patients with hysterical amnesia. Such patients can often, but by no means always, retrieve repressed memories for past events and give reasonable accounts of relevant portions of their past history. The interview can be used both in patients with isolated episodes of amnesia, as for example for episodes of rape or assault or murder, or for patients who profess total amnesia for their entire past lives. Amobarbital given intravenously also is occasionally effective in resolving hysterical paralyses and other conversion symptoms.

Intravenous amobarbital also has a remarkable property in many patients in psychotic stupor. Although the stupor used to be generally referred to as catatonic stupor, there is currently some doubt whether individual cases of psychic mutism with frozen motor behavior are in fact a manifestation of schizophrenia or a manifestation of psychotic depression. In either case, intravenous amobarbital given as in an Amytal interview can often produce a remarkable change in a patient's behavior. The frozen stupor will often clear remarkably, and the patient will be able to talk spontaneously, walk about, drink fluids, eat a meal, and otherwise carry on apparently normal activity for a half hour or sometimes for two to three hours. In some patients the psychotic material suppressed by the stupor becomes blatantly obvious as the patient talks about the delusions, hallucinations, and bizarre preoccupations. In other cases, the patient appears really quite normal without unusual thought content. Such patients often have no idea of why their behavior has become frozen and immobilized and why they are unable to speak or move. Obviously, the Amytal interview can occasionally be useful in the rare cases where a mute catatonic patient has been admitted to an emergency room or a psychiatric unit with no history and no identification and the clinician is unable to decide even what the patient's name and address are, much less what the past history or probably psychiatric diagnosis is. In such situations, amobarbital given intravenously can be quite helpful in clarifying the situation. However, it should only be administered after all reasonable medical or pharmacological causes for such a mute or unresponsive state have been ruled out.

MEPROBAMATE

Meprobamate occupies an intermediate position between the benzodiazepines and the barbiturates, both pharmacologically and historically. It was first marketed about 1956,

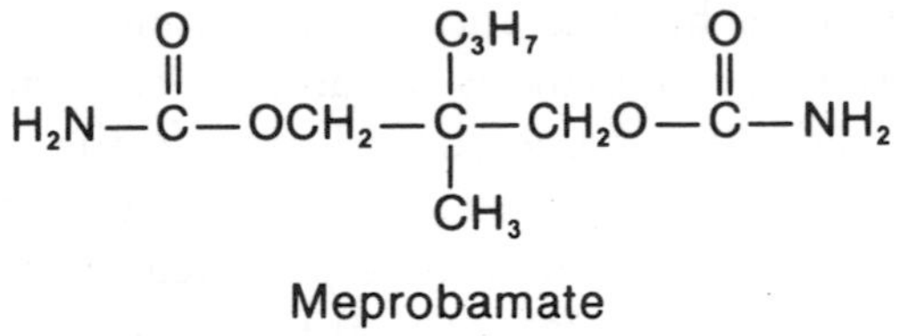

$$H_2N-\overset{\displaystyle O}{\overset{\|}{C}}-OCH_2-\overset{\displaystyle C_3H_7}{\underset{\displaystyle CH_3}{\overset{|}{\underset{|}{C}}}}-CH_2O-\overset{\displaystyle O}{\overset{\|}{C}}-NH_2$$

Meprobamate

Figure 6-3. Chemical Structure of Meprobamate

having evolved from a chemically related muscle relaxant named mephenesin. Its structure is shown in Figure 6-3. Meprobamate has muscle relaxant and sedative properties, but it was initially evaluated as an antianxiety agent. On the basis of a small number of enthusiastic but uncontrolled studies in anxiety, it was released to the market in the days when the Food and Drug Administration required only evidence of safety rather than evidence of efficacy. It became an instant national success with widespread publicity in the lay media.

Now that the dust has settled, 20 years later, it is clear that meprobamate is, in fact, an effective antianxiety agent in the same sense that diazepam or chlordiazepoxide are effective, although controlled studies directly comparing the efficacy of meprobamate with benzodiazepines are almost nonexistent. The clinical dose of meprobamate is on the order of 400 mg three or four times a day, being approximately equivalent to 5 mg of diazepam three or four times a day (Table 6-C). The major side effects are sedation and malcoordination. The drug is relatively safe in overdose, less lethal than intermediate acting barbiturates like pentobarbital, but a good deal less safe than diazepam. The drug produces physical dependence and tolerance in much the same way as do the barbiturates and the benzodiazepines. Significant withdrawal effects such as convulsions, agitation, or delirium occur after clinically relatively lower doses of meprobamate, for example, after 3200 mg or eight 400 mg pills a day.

Currently, it is hard to identify any unique advantages possessed by meprobamate as an antianxiety drug. Among possible considerations one should include the fact that it has been widely manufactured generically and therefore may be an inexpensive alternative to a patented benzodiazepine such as alprazolam or lorazepam. It is a reasonably effective and reasonably satisfactory hypnotic at a dose of 400-800 mg a day at bedtime. Clinically, we have seen occasional anxious patients who have a marked subjective intolerance to benzodiazepines becoming agitated, dysphoric, and restless on any of several of them. Some of these patients tolerate meprobamate quite well. It can also be used in such rare patients for whom an antianxiety drug is to be prescribed during the daytime, either as a prn medication or for four to six weeks. To our knowledge no one has evaluated meprobamate in such conditions as akathisia or panic disorder where benzodiazepines may or may not be effective.

Deprol, a 30-year-old meprobamate-containing combination medication, deserves mention here. This combination of benactyzine and meprobamate is still marketed for use in depression. Each tablet contains 400 mg of meprobamate and 1 mg of benactyzine hydrochloride. There is essentially no evidence that benactyzine by itself is an effective antidepressant, although the compound is anticholinergic and might conceivably have some antidepressant properties. One trial in schizophrenic patients made many years ago shows benactyzine to increase hallucinatory and psychotic behavior. However, there are a handful of studies suggesting that Deprol is effective in some depressions and perhaps more effective than either of its ingredients. The question remains moot, and we have not heard of the compound being used clinically for a number of years.

NORADRENERGIC AGENTS

In recent years, a number of studies have pointed to the potential use of beta blockers (e.g., propranolol) and primarily presynaptic but also postsynaptic alpha$_2$ receptor agonists (e.g., clonidine) to ameliorate symptoms of anxiety. Use of these agents stems from the observations that certain symptoms (e.g., palpitations, sweating, etc.) of anxiety suggest involvement of the sympathetic nervous system. Investigations were first directed toward the use of beta blockers in anxious musical performers. A number of years later, clonidine was shown by Gold et al. (1978) to be effective in blocking physiologic symptoms associated with opioid withdrawal, resulting in its eventual application to patients with anxiety disorders and recently those in nicotine withdrawal. This drug exerts alpha$_2$ (presynaptic) receptor agonist effects; however, since it is also a postsynaptic alpha$_2$ agonist, its pharmacologic actions are complex.

Clinical Indications, Names, and Structures

Beta blockers (e.g., propranolol) are indicated for hypertension, prophylaxis against angina, arrhythmias, migraine headaches, and hypertrophic subaortic stenosis. They are not FDA approved for "use" in anxiety, although several studies suggest propranolol may be useful. These studies were originally conducted in Great Britain and point to beta blockers having particularly potent effects on the somatic manifestations of anxiety (e.g., palpitations, tremors, etc.) with less dramatic effects noted on the psychic component of anxiety. The antitremor properties of these drugs have resulted in their being commonly used in patients in whom hand tremors have developed secondary to lithium carbonate (see Chapter 5). More recently a number of reports have suggested that although beta blockers have some use in generalized anxiety, they are not particularly effective in blocking panic attacks. Indeed Gorman et al. (1983) reported that propranolol failed to block lactate-induced panic attacks. However, some investigators have noted that propranolol may block panic anxiety resulting from isoproterenol (an adrenergic agonist) infusions and thus could still be effective in some patients with panic attacks.

Clonidine has an FDA indication for the treatment of hypertension. As noted above, it has been widely studied and used for blocking physiologic symptoms of opioid withdrawal (e.g., palpitations, sweating, etc.). The drug has also been studied in anxiety and in panic disorder and has been shown to be effective in both, although tolerance frequently develops to the antianxiety effects. It is conceivable that the drug's mixed, partial pre- and postsynaptic receptor agonist properties may enter into the development of tolerance. Clonidine has also been used to test various aspects of the catecholamine hypotheses of affective and anxiety disorders. (Generic and trade names of key noradrenergic agents are summarized in Table 6-C.)

Dosage Ranges

Using propranolol as a model, clinicians should begin patients with peripheral symptoms of anxiety or with lithium-induced tremor at 10 mg BID and increase incrementally to approximately 80-160 mg/day (see Table 6-C). Although the usual maintenance dosage of the drug in patients with hypertension is as high as 240 mg/day, such dosages are rarely needed for anxious or tremulous patients. Generally, the use of these agents in patients with anxiety disorders should parallel that of the benzodiazepines, with attempts made at trying patients off the drug after a few weeks of treatment. In tremors secondary to lithium carbonate, many patients show a reemergence of their tremors after discontinuation of the beta blocker, resulting in their remaining on beta blockers for prolonged periods. We know of no major untoward effects that have resulted; however, since some patients may become lethargic and even depressed on beta blockers, clinicians need to keep this in mind in patients with a major affective disorder (see below). This is a confusing area since we have also used propranolol for tricyclic-induced tremor without affecting the depression in the vast majority of patients.

Clonidine should be started at a dose of 0.1 mg BID and increased by 0.1 mg every one to two days to a total daily dose of 0.4-0.6 mg (Table 6-C). Since some studies have indicated that tolerance develops to this drug, clinicians should attempt to limit the duration of exposure to these drugs whenever possible.

Side Effects

Side effects of the beta blockers include bradycardia, hypotension, weakness, fatigue, clouded sensorium, gastrointestinal upset, and bronchospasm, among others. For the psychiatrist, a few particular caveats appear warranted. Clinicians need to remember that these drugs are contraindicated in asthmatics because they may produce bronchospasm and in patients with Reynaud's disease because of the risk of increased peripheral vasoconstriction. As for their capacity to cause depression, we have not seen patients who have developed true depressive disorders. Rather, we have noted that some patients may feel "washed out" or lethargic. However, clinicians at other institutions have reported cases of propranolol-induced depression with endogenous features that remit with discontinuation of the drug. When stopping beta blockers, it is wisest to taper the dose to avoid any rebound phenomena that could result in untoward cardiac or blood pressure effects.

Clonidine also has a relatively favorable side-effect profile. Its major side effects include dry mouth, fatigue, and hypotension. In hypertensive patients BID scheduling (with two-thirds of the dose given at sleep) has been advocated to deal with its sedating effects. Discontinuation should be gradual to avoid rebound or the hypertensive crises that have been reported in hypertensive patients who were suddenly withdrawn from the drug.

ANTIDEPRESSANTS AS ANXIOLYTIC AGENTS

Agoraphobia and Panic

Several antidepressants exert major antianxiety effects. Imipramine was first reported by Klein and colleagues in the 1960s to have potent anxiolytic effects in agoraphobic patients with panic. Clinically, it appears that most, if not all, TCAs exert similar antipanic effects. In addition the MAOI phenelzine is also a potent antipanic agent as are probably the other MAOIs and trazodone. However, not all antidepressants are antipanic drugs. Most notably, bupropion appears not to exert antipanic effects. The noradrenergic effects of various antidepressants (particularly the TCAs and MAOIs) on the locus ceruleus generally have been invoked to explain their antipanic activity. Whether this explains the possible antipanic effects of trazodone is unclear. Bupropion exerts little or no effect on noradrenergic systems.

Early on, the general rule of thumb was that panic patients required only low doses of TCAs (e.g., 50 mg/day of imipramine) to respond. In the past few years, it has become more evident that, as in depression, many panic patients require relatively higher doses of TCAs or MAOIs, although a small proportion are very sensitive to TCAs, tolerating only 10-25 mg of imipramine a day. We recommend using the general dosage regimens of TCAs in depression (see Chapter 3).

Generalized Anxiety Disorder

Recently, collaborative studies have pointed out that TCAs also exert effects in generalized anxiety disorder. In one major study, imipramine was as effective at four to six weeks as the benzodiazepine chlordiazepoxide in patients with this disorder. However, in the first two weeks, the benzodiazepine was more effective. Given the need for rapid improvement and the greater side effects with TCAs, the TCAs should not be viewed as first-line drugs in generalized anxiety disorder. They can be used in patients who do not respond quickly to benzodiazepines.

Obsessive-Compulsive Disorder

A small number of case reports in the literature describe favorable responses in obsessive-compulsive patients being treated with almost any available medications, including antipsychotic drugs, lithium, tricyclic drugs, and MAOIs. All of these probably work in occasional patients, although one would guess that antipsychotic drugs are more helpful in schizophrenic patients with marked obsessive-compulsive features, and drugs commonly used in depression are most effective in alleviating secondary depression when it is superimposed upon the obsessive-compulsive disorder itself.

However, there is a large battery of clinical lore from Europe and from individual practitioners in the United States that asserts that clomipramine (Anafranil) is substantially better than all other drug therapies in obsessive-compulsive disorder. Insel et al. (1983) at NIMH carried out consecutive open studies of clomipramine, desipramine, and zimelidine and reported clomipramine to be most effective, zimelidine somewhat effective, and desipramine ineffective. A large double-blind study comparing clomipramine with imipramine in obsessive-compulsive disorder was completed in the United States a few years ago but has not been published to date. The results are said to have shown that the two drugs both cause essentially equivalent amounts of improvement in the first four weeks. In the second four weeks clomipramine was significantly superior to imipramine in causing further improvement. This alleged finding conforms to Insel's experience and the clinical impressions of many psychopharmacologists.

Clomipramine causes gradual and progressive improvement in obsessive-compulsive symptoms, more impressive in the second month of treatment than in the first.

Clomipramine, therefore, may well be the drug of choice in obsessive-compulsive disorder. The drug's marketing in the United States is delayed because of differences of opinion between the company and the Food and Drug Administration over the available evidence as to the drug's efficacy. The drug can now be obtained under complex conditions from CIBA-Geigy for humanitarian use if each individual psychiatrist will file with the FDA for permission to use clomipramine as an investigational drug for each specific patient.

Clomipramine is a potent serotonin reuptake blocker, and this action has been proposed to underlie the anti-obsessive-compulsive effect. However, the drug is demethylated in humans, and the resultant metabolite is a potent norepinephrine reuptake blocker. Since some obsessive-compulsive patients respond to other antidepressants, it seems reasonable to first prescribe a more serotonergic antidepressant (amitriptyline or trazodone first and then an MAOI) before seeking a trial on clomipramine, if available.

ANTIHISTAMINES

The antihistamine hydroxyzine enjoys indications for the treatment of anxiety and tension associated with psychoneurotic conditions or physical disease states. It is also indicated in the treatment of pruritis due to allergic conditions and for pre- and postoperative sedation. In psychiatric practice these drugs are less commonly used in treating anxious patients, reflecting their less potent anxiolytic effects.

Hydroxyzine's recommended oral dosage in adults is 50-100 mg QID (Table 6-C). The major side effects include drowsiness and dry mouth. It does not produce physical dependence. It may produce central nervous system depression when added to alcohol, narcotic analgesics, central

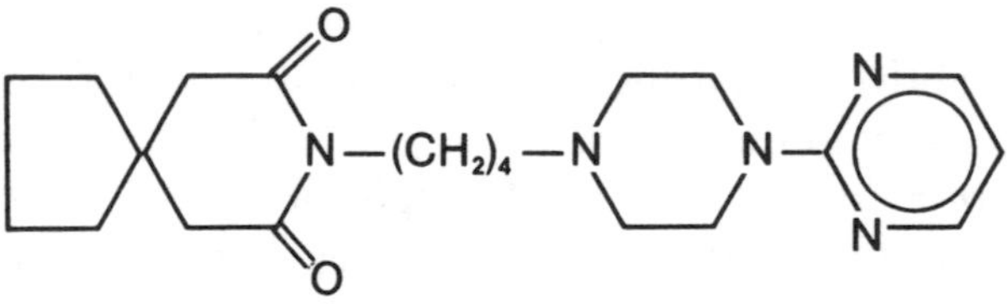

Buspirone

Figure 6-4. Chemical Structure of Buspirone

nervous system depressants, and tricyclic antidepressants. The antihistamine diphenhydramine is commonly used in medicine and psychiatry as a sedative/hypnotic. Its use is described in Chapter 7.

BUSPIRONE

The development of buspirone—a nonbenzodiazepine, generally nonsedating anxiolytic—has stirred considerable excitement in psychopharmacologic circles. It represents the first prominent anxiolytic to be introduced since the benzodiazepines. The drug was originally developed as a potential antipsychotic agent. However, it was found in early clinical trials to have little antipsychotic potency but was eventually shown to have antiaggression effects in primates and antianxiety effects in humans. Buspirone will have the brand name of Buspar. Its structure is shown in Figure 6-4.

The drug does not bind with high affinity to benzodiazepine and GABA receptors, although it may have an effect on the chloride channel coupled to the benzodiazepine/GABA complex. Buspirone has little antiseizure effect. Its anxiolytic effects have been postulated to be via dopaminergic properties, although the drug's central effects are not entirely clear. Some investigators have argued that buspirone exerts potent presynaptic dopamine antagonist effects resulting in increased dopamine at the synapses. Others have noted that the drug also has peripheral postsynaptic dopamine blocking properties. Recently, buspirone has also been reported to exert effects on serotonin systems.

The apparent advantages of buspirone lie in its not being sedating at the usual anxiolytic dosages and having little potential for addiction or abuse. Obviously, wider clinical use will ultimately provide the answers as to the drug's potential untoward effects. The drug has been compared with and found to be as effective as traditional benzodiazepines under double-blind conditions in the treatment of patients with generalized anxiety disorder. It has, to date, not been fully studied in patients with panic disorder, and efficacy in this condition is unclear.

The dosage of buspirone is similar to that of diazepam. The average daily dosage is 15-25 mg/day with an initial dose of 5 mg BID. At single doses of 20-40 mg/day, the drug produces sedation or dysphoria. It probably can be administered chronically instead of the benzodiazepines in generalized anxiety disorder; however, most such studies have been of such relatively short duration (about four weeks) that further data are required.

Side effects include headache, nausea, dizziness, and tension, which generally are not major problems. Indeed, the drug appears to have a more desirable side effect profile than do the benzodiazepines. It does not appear to impair motor coordination and shows little untoward interaction with alcohol. According to Sathanathan et al. (1975), the drug may exacerbate psychosis in schizoaffective patients, reflecting complex prodopaminergic properties.

Two additional potential problems or limitations come to mind as this drug is being introduced. For one, it may not block symptoms associated with benzodiazepine withdrawal. Clinicians should keep this in mind if they are considering switching a patient from a benzodiazepine to buspirone. Traditional gradual reduction of the benzodiazepine may be required. A second problem revolves around whether the drug will cause (or relieve) extrapyramidal symptoms in some patients. The drug's complex central dopaminergic effects could result in unexpected side reactions when the drug is in wider clinical use. Overall to date, buspirone must be viewed as one of the exciting steps forward in the treatment of patients with anxiety disorders.

Bibliography

Braestrup C, Squires RF: Brain specific benzodiazepine receptors. Br J Psychiatry 133:249–260, 1978

Buspirone: A new generation anxiolytic. International Drug Therapy Newsletter 19:1–4, 1984

Gold MS, Redmond DE Jr, Kleber HD: Clonidine in opiate withdrawal. Lancet 1:929–930, 1978

Goldberg HL, Finnerty RJ: The comparative efficacy of buspirone and diazepam in the treatment of anxiety. Am J Psychiatry 126:1184–1187, 1979

Goldberg HL: Buspirone hydrochloride: a unique new anxiolytic agent. Pharmacokinetics, clinical pharmacology, abuse potential and clinical efficacy. Pharmacotherapy 4:315–324, 1984

Gorman JM, Levy GF, Liebowitz MR, et al: Effect of acute beta-adrenergic blockade or lactate induced panic. Arch Gen Psychiatry 40:1079–1082, 1983

Granville-Grossman KL, Turner P: The effect of propranolol on anxiety. Lancet 1:788–790, 1966

Greenblatt DJ, Shader RI, Abernethy DR: Current status of benzodiazepines [first of two parts]. N Engl J Med 309:354–359, 1983

Greenblatt DJ, Shader RI, Abernethy DR: Current status of benzodiazepines [second of two parts]. N Engl J Med 309:410–415, 1983

Grinker R, Spiegel J: Men under stress. Philadelphia, Blakiston, 1945

Insel TR, Murphy DL, Cohen RM, et al: Obsessive compulsive disorder: a double-blind trial of clomipramine and clorgyline. Arch Gen Psychiatry 40:605–612, 1983

Insel TR (ed): New Findings in Obsessive-Compulsive Disorder. Washington, DC, American Psychiatric Press, 1984

Isbell H, Altschul S, Kornetsky C, et al: Chronic barbiturate intoxication: an experimental study. AMA Archives of Neurology and Psychiatry 64:1–28, 1950

Kahn R, McNair D, Covi L, et al: Effects of psychotropic agents in high anxiety subjects. Psychopharmacol Bull 17:97–100, 1981

Klein DF: Importance of psychiatric diagnosis in prediction of clinical drug effects. Arch Gen Psychiatry 16:118–126, 1967

Lader M: Summary and commentary, in Pharmacology of Benzodiazepines. Edited by Usdin E, Skolnick P, Tallman JF, et al. New York, Macmillan, 1982, pp 53–60

Liebowitz MR, Fyer AJ, McGrath P, et al: Clonidine treatment of panic disorder. Psychopharmacol Bull 17:122–123, 1981

Lucki I, Rickels K, Geller AM: Chronic use of benzodiazepines and cognitive test performance. Psychopharmacology (in press)

Meltzer HY, Fleming R, Robertson A: The effect of buspirone on prolactin and growth hormone secretion in man. Arch Gen Psychiatry 40:1099–1102, 1983

Mooney JJ, Schatzberg AF, Cole JO, et al: Enhanced signal transduction by adenylate cyclase in platelet membranes of patients showing antidepressant responses to alprazolam: preliminary data. J Psychiatr Res 19:65–75, 1985

Noyes R, Anderson DJ, Clancy J, et al: Diazepam and propranolol in panic disorder and agoraphobia. Arch Gen Psychiatry 41:287–292, 1984

Ribbet LA, Eison AS, Eison MA, et al: Neuropharmacology of buspirone. Psychopathology 17(Suppl 3):69–78, 1984

Rickels K, Chase WG, Downing RW: Long-term diazepam therapy and clinical outcome. JAMA 250:767–771, 1983

Sathananthan GL, Sanzhavi F, Phillips N: MJ 9022 (buspirone): Correlation between neuroleptic potential and stereotypy. Current Therapeutic Research 18:701–705, 1975

Sethy VH: Pharmacokinetic studies of triazolobenzodiazepines by drug-receptor binding assays, in Pharmacology of Benzodiazepines. Edited by Usdin E, Skolnick P, Tallman JF, et al. New York, Macmillan, 1982

Sheehan DV, Ballenger J, Jacobsen G: Treatment of endogenous anxiety with phobic, hysterical, and hypochondriacal symptoms. Arch Gen Psychiatry 37:51–59, 1980

Sheehan DV, Davidson J, Manshreck TC, et al: Lack of efficacy of a new antidepressant (bupropion) in the treatment of panic disorder with phobias. J Clin Psychopharmacol 3:23–31, 1983

Sheehan DV: Some biochemical correlates of panic attack with agoraphobia and their response to a new treatment. J Clin Psychopharmacol 4:66–75, 1984

Skolnick P, Paul SM, Weissman BA: Preclinical pharmacology of buspirone hydrochloride. Pharmacotherapy 4:308–314, 1984

Tyrer PJ, Lader MH: Clinical response to propranolol and diazepam in somatic and psychic anxiety. Br Med J 2:14–16, 1974

Zitrin CM, Klein DF, Woerner MG: Treatment of phobias, I: Comparison of imipramine hydrochloride and placebo. Arch Gen Psychiatry 40:125–138, 1983

Hypnotics

7

Insomnia is a common and troubling enough problem for many patients to seek help from psychiatrists or sleep disorder specialists. Many patients complain, often despairingly, of very poor sleep or total insomnia, but nevertheless appear on all-night sleep recordings or nurses' or relatives' observations to be sleeping most of the night. Attempts to objectify insomnia in terms of the time it takes for the person to fall asleep or the length of time actually slept have often not proven useful. Also, the psychiatrist is not uncommonly faced with patients who are actually awake all night, particularly those with marked depression and anxiety, whose sleep is so disturbed that they feel exhausted the next day and claim that they "can't function."

In psychiatric patients, troublesome insomnia is often one feature of a wider symptom complex, which may also include diurnal rhythm disturbances of activity, mood, etc. Depressed patients classically have early morning awakening and diurnal variation. Some, however, have marked difficulty falling asleep as well. Patients with pronounced initial insomnia may be separated into those who sleep fitfully and poorly even after falling asleep and those who do sleep well after even several hours of initial insomnia. Such patients can sleep from 4:00 A.M. until noon. A few patients with very severe depression complain of almost complete insomnia, claiming they lie in bed all night without sleeping, often experiencing dysphoric, miserable ruminations.

Other psychiatric conditions are also manifested by sleep disturbances. Patients with anxiety disorders are more likely to have trouble falling asleep. Those with mania or hypomania may stay up all night either happily overactive or dysphorically agitated, as may patients with schizophrenia or schizophreniform psychoses. Classically, manic patients do not complain of sleeplessness but rather claim that they do not *need* to sleep. Demented organic patients may become more confused and agitated toward evening (sundowner syndrome) and may also be agitated at night after having slept all day. Patients very upset by major stress—bereavement, rejections, physical trauma—may have insomnia as part of an acute stress response.

Insomnia in all of the relatively acute psychiatric conditions mentioned above is fairly straightforward to treat. Insomnia as part of a depressive disorder almost always responds to a standard antidepressant—in fact, some of the more sedative tricyclics (amitriptyline, doxepin, trimipramine) may be useful hypnotics even in the absence of depression. For depression with poor sleep, it is sensible to begin with a sedative tricyclic (see Chapter 3), but even more stimulant tricyclics such as protriptyline or desipramine usually improve sleep as the depressive syndrome improves. In manic and schizophrenic excitements and in some organic agitations, the insomnia responds well to antipsychotic drugs of any class, although chlorpromazine and thioridazine may initially be slightly more effective as hypnotics before the general syndrome ameliorates.

Thus, the best general approach is to treat the psychiatric

condition that underlies the insomnia with drugs that are appropriate to that condition rather than prescribing a benzodiazepine or other hypnotic drug first for the insomnia and then treating the depression or psychosis later.

In principle, a psychiatrist can run an inpatient ward or treat outpatients without ever prescribing a hypnotic. In practice, however, life often is (or appears to be) more complicated. Other patients, families, and nursing staff members become very upset if patients do not retire to bed and sleep without disturbing them. Often, hypnotics end up being prescribed to cut down on distress in the patient and his or her milieu. Such prescribing is often justifiable but can pose problems. First, the hypnotic may not put the patient to sleep but instead may leave the patient groggy, confused, and even more agitated. Second, a long-acting hypnotic, like flurazepam, may leave the patient groggy the next day. Third, once the patient is used to getting a hypnotic (and the doctor is used to prescribing it), the practice may continue for weeks or even months, long after the initial phase of the illness or the stress of hospitalization is past. When the sleeping pill is finally stopped, rebound insomnia is likely to occur and lead to resumption of the hypnotic to control it.

Another problem is the new patient being admitted to the hospital (or visiting a new psychiatrist) who is thoroughly accustomed to taking, for months or years, 60 mg of flurazepam or 2000 mg of chloral hydrate at bedtime but who still complains of poor sleep, which is, of course, reportedly much worse if the hypnotic is stopped. Here, the obvious options are to taper the hypnotic gradually while treating the major psychiatric disorder or to continue it while dealing with the core condition. The difficulty with the second, interpersonally easier, option is that the hypnotic may never actually be discontinued. A more complicated version of this scenario is the patient who comes to the psychiatrist while on several psychoactive drugs of different classes, all of which need to be withdrawn or changed. In this situation, it is common to leave the hypnotic at a stable dose and taper and stop the other drugs first to avoid confusing the effects of stopping the hypnotic with the already potentially complex effects of also discontinuing a tricyclic antidepressant or an antipsychotic.

At present, the only real indications for hypnotics in insomnia are for brief (three- to seven-day) use or occasional use in transitory insomnia caused either by acute life stresses or by major shifts in diurnal rhythm, as in jet lag or changing from one work shift to another.

Although it is wise to avoid prolonged hypnotic usage, prolonged use of a benzodiazepine hypnotic may be less harmful than is often said and may in fact provide some benefit. The available evidence from sleep laboratories suggests that hypnotics improve sleep measurably for only about a week, but many confirmed hypnotic users swear that the hypnotics are *always* helpful and even vitally necessary. Perhaps the initial sedation at peak blood level provides a familiar conditioned cue conducive to falling asleep. Certainly, some patients who have taken hypnotics every night for several years continue to complain of poor sleep and daytime fatigue and dysphoria for months after the hypnotic has been stopped. A sleep expert can often prove helpful in the treatment of chronic insomnia with persistent hypnotic dependence by using behavioral techniques.

Some patients who present to psychiatrists may actually suffer from a primary sleep disorder or have a sleep disorder secondary to medications. In patients in whom insomnia is a major or primary complaint, sleep apnea should be considered as a diagnosis, especially if snoring with irregular respiration is noted by the patient's bedmate. Nocturnal myoclonus may result in extremely disturbed sleep characterized by thrashing about. The condition often responds to 1-3 mg of clonazepam at bedtime. Narcolepsy on occasion will present as atypical depression with fatigue and hypersomnia and can be treated with stimulants and perhaps protriptyline. On the other hand, excessive intake of stimulants—caffeine and diet pills, as well as phenylpropanolamine used in treatment of sinus disorders, cough, or asthma—may cause insomnia. Hyperthyroidism is also a frequent cause of insomnia.

Insomnia, often quite troublesome, can also occur as a complication of psychotropic therapy. Some patients develop insomnia if stimulant tricyclics (desipramine and protriptyline) are given at bedtime, and a few patients even develop insomnia on all—or many—tricyclics, including amitriptyline. Our experience has been that doxepin or trimipramine is more likely to be tolerated by such patients. Sometimes moving the tricyclic from bedtime administration to daytime will resolve this problem.

The MAOIs can produce severe insomnia in patients showing an otherwise excellent response. Often this insomnia is not initially bothersome; however, some patients do become very troubled by a reduction of sleep of four or more hours. Shifting the dose to early in the day usually does not help. These patients may require hypnotics or low-dose amitriptyline (see Chapter 3).

HYPNOTIC BENZODIAZEPINES

The benzodiazepines are the most widely prescribed sedative/ hypnotics in the United States today. For many years, only one benzodiazepine (flurazepam) enjoyed an indication as a hypnotic, although most benzodiazepines have hypnotic properties. In the past few years, two new hypnotic benzodiazepines have become available—temazepam and triazolam.

The principles for discriminating among these three drugs are similar to those described in Chapter 6 for the anxiolytic benzodiazepines—structure, pharmacokinetics, absorption, and distribution (Table 7-A). For example, each of these hypnotics belongs to a separate structural subclass: 2-keto-

Table 7-A. Hypnotic Benzodiazepines

Generic Name	Brand Name	Dosage Form	Dosage (mg/day)	Absorption	Major Active Components	Approximate Half-Life (hours)
flurazepam	Dalmane	Capsules: 15/30 mg	15–30	intermediate	hydroxyethyl flurazepam desalkylflurazepam	1 100
temazepam	Restoril	Capsules: 15/30 mg	15–30	intermediate to slow	temazepam	9
triazolam	Halcion	Tablets: 0.125/ 0.25/0.5 mg	0.125–0.5	intermediate	triazolam	3

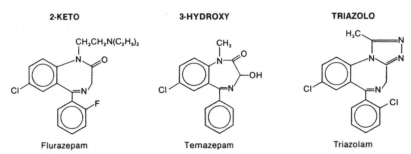

Figure 7-1. Chemical Structures of Hypnotic Benzodiazepines

(flurazepam), 3-OH- (temazepam), and triazolo- (triazolam) (Figure 7-1).

The metabolism and half-lives of these subclass members parallel their anxiolytic counterparts. Flurazepam is oxidized in the liver and, like diazepam, it has a relatively long half-life (40 hours) and also forms a long-acting (100 hours) metabolite, desalkyflurazepam. Temazepam is conjugated with a glucuronide radical in the liver and has a much shorter half-life (eight hours) and has no active metabolites. Triazolam is oxidized but with no clearly active metabolites and enjoys an extremely short half-life (three to six hours) (Table 7-A).

The absorption of flurazepam and triazolam are more rapid (peak blood levels occur at 30 and 20 minutes, respectively) than that of temazepam, which may not be absorbed for 45-60 minutes. The slower absorption accounts for patients not falling asleep rapidly after taking this medication. Clinicians should advise patients to take temazepam approximately one hour before retiring to avoid anticipatory discomfort and their resorting to premature repeat dosing.

The distribution of the sedative benzodiazepines is relatively rapid. Indeed, the acute formation of high peak blood levels is thought to account for why patients fall asleep relatively quickly on these drugs. The decline from peak levels may account for why patients can awaken often, even when they still show significant drug plasma levels. Moreover, the decline from peak levels and the need for peak levels to induce sleep also explain why patients treated with longer acting benzodiazepines like flurazepam require nightly dosages.

Some investigators and clinicians have argued that the new shorter acting compounds (particularly temazepam) offer great advantages since they are largely excreted by the next morning. Indeed, a recent study points to the safe use of triazolam for inducing sleep on transatlantic flights and preventing jet lag. However, as discussed above, there may be disadvantages associated with shorter acting hypnotics— particularly rebound insomnia. Rebound insomnia represents a worsening of sleep disturbance occurring soon after discontinuing the hypnotic. With the short-acting hypnotics, this occurs within the first two nights after discontinuation and can be troublesome for patients. Although acutely apparent with shorter acting compounds, it may occur after five to seven days of discontinuation of benzodiazepines with longer half-lives and may be misinterpreted as a reemergence of the underlying insomnia rather than as a rebound phenomenon. When rebound insomnia occurs, clinicians should avoid resumption of the drug. Rather, reassurance and the prescription of antihistaminic sedatives (e.g., 50 mg of diphenhydramine) for a few days may prove beneficial. In cases where this does not work, reinstituting the benzodiazepine and gradually tapering the dose is an alternative strategy.

The side effects of the sedative hypnotic benzodiazepines are similar to those of their anxiolytic counterparts. They include sedation, ataxia, anterograde amnesia, slurred speech, and nausea. These side effects are not particularly dangerous, although sedation can be a problem if the individual attempts to drive, operates heavy machinery, etc. There is weak evidence to suggest that the longer half-life compounds cause clinically important cognitive problems the following day; however, this area has not been well studied. Refined and detailed psychological testing can usually detect impairment of cognitive or psychomotor function the morning after a benzodiazepine hypnotic has been used to induce sleep. The real question is whether this impairment is clinically important; the vast majority of hypnotic users do not note behavioral impairment the next day unless they also note persisting sedation as well.

BARBITURATES

A number of barbiturates enjoy FDA indications for usage as sedative hypnotics. These compounds are listed in Table 7-B. Pentobarbital, secobarbital, amobarbital, and a combination of secobarbital and amobarbital are those most commonly used for nighttime sedation. In addition, several of these enjoy indications for both day and nighttime sedation. (The use of amobarbital, butisol, and other barbiturates for daytime sedation is discussed in Chapter 6.) Dosage ranges of these compounds and routes of administration are also listed in Table 7-B. Structures are shown in Figure 6-2.

For many years barbiturates were widely used for their hypnotic effects, but their use has dwindled with the introduction of the safer benzodiazepines. The half-lives of barbiturates determine their clinical applications. The extremely short-acting barbiturates (e.g., hexobarbital) are used for preanesthesia or anesthesia. Intermediate-duration barbiturates (e.g., pentobarbital) are used for induction and maintenance of sleep. Longer acting compounds may be used for agitation or anxiety (see Chapter 6). Barbiturate preparations are variations of a barbituric acid structure with substitutions at one or more key positions, resulting in differences in lipophilia and half-lives (see Figure 6-2).

The barbiturates have become less widely used because of their limited safety margin in overdosage, potential for dependence, and the degree of central nervous system depression they induce. These drugs are extremely potent hypnotics, particularly for patients who have not previously

Table 7-B. Barbiturates for Insomnia

Generic Name	Brand Name	Dosage Forms	Nighttime Dosage (mg)*
amobarbital	Amytal	Tablets: 15/30/50/100 mg Concentrate: 44 mg/5 ml (16 oz bottles)	160–200
	Amytal Sodium	Capsules: 65/200 mg Vials: 250/500 mg	65–200
aprobarbital	Atarate	Concentrate: 40 mg/5 ml (16 oz bottles)	5–20 ml
butabarbital	Buticaps	Capsules: 15/30 mg	50–100
	Butisol Sodium	Capsules: 15/30/50/100 mg Concentrate: 30 mg/5 ml (16 oz bottles)	50–100
pentobarbital	Nembutal	Capsules: 30/50/100 mg Concentrate: 20 mg/5 ml (16 oz bottles)	100
		Parenteral: 50 mg/ml (2 ml ampules, 20 and 50 ml vials)	150–200
		Suppositories: 30/60/120/ 200 mg	120–200
pheno-barbital	Generic	Capsules: 16 mg 65 mg (sustained release) Tablets: 8/15/16/30/32/65/ 100 mg Concentrate: 16 mg/ml drops, 20 mg/5 ml	100–320
		Parenteral: multiple strengths	100–320
secobarbital	Seconal	Capsules: 50/100 mg Parenteral: 50 mg/ml (20 ml vials)	100
		Suppositories: 30/60/120/ 200 mg	30–200
secobarbital and amo-barbital	Tuinal	Combinations of 25/50/ 100 mg each	50–200

* Adult dosages. For child dosages, consult *PDR* or similar reference.

taken barbiturates. Indeed, some patients may demonstrate considerable somnolesence 24 hours after ingestion. Moreover, these agents pose potential problems when mixed with alcohol or other central nervous system depressants and are contraindicated in patients with acute intermittent porphyria.

In depressed patients, the administration of barbiturates may result in a marked reduction of tricyclic antidepressant plasma levels and diminutions of antidepressant effects because of their induction of liver microsomal enzymes and accelerated degradation of the tricyclic. Clinicians should keep this in mind when considering adjunctive usage of hypnotics in depressed patients. Indeed, we have seen depressed patients who had chronically been on barbiturates for sleep fail to respond to amitriptyline and other tricyclics but who did respond after discontinuing their barbiturates.

At present the main remaining use in outpatient psychiatry for intermediate-acting sedative-hypnotic barbiturates, such as pentobarbital, is probably limited to the older patient who occasionally needs a hypnotic for insomnia and, because of prolonged past experience with barbiturates, finds a barbiturate sleeping pill preferable to any of the newer benzodiazepines. Such prescribing is of course a matter of giving in to a patient's experience and preference rather than a mandatory or necessary clinical maneuver. (For discussion of various uses of amobarbital—including for analytically oriented interviews—the reader is referred to Chapter 6.)

For patients who have become dependent on barbiturates, detoxification is necessary. Abrupt withdrawal should be avoided because it can result in seizures, delirium, and even death. When the daily dose of barbiturate is not known, physicians can give test doses of a barbiturate (watching for the emergence of nystagmus, slurred speech, ataxia, and sedation) to determine the currently needed dosage. This can then act as a barometer of the dose at which to begin a detoxification program (see Chapter 11).

SEDATIVE ANTIHISTAMINES

Hydroxyzine compounds are the only antihistamines with some documented efficacy in the treatment of anxiety disorders. They also enjoy indication for preoperative and postanesthesia sedation. These drugs are available in capsules or tablets ranging all the way from 10 to 100 mg each. However, our clinical experience in psychiatric patients suggests that these drugs are neither much appreciated by patients nor particularly effective on the few occasions when it has been tried by us. They are reasonably free of side effects, although hydroxyzine and the other antihistamines exert anticholinergic effects. When taken with other anticholinergic agents, hydroxyzine and related compounds can pose potential problems, particularly in high dosages. They may mainly have value as a delaying action for patients who are inclined to abuse sedative hypnotic or benzodiazepine drugs, since they do not produce either physical or psychic dependence.

Diphenhydramine (Benadryl) is another antihistamine that is sometimes used for its sedative or alleged hypnotic effects. It has not been well studied in either capacity but has some sedative properties and is occasionally judged by patients to be acceptable. Dosage for sleep is 50-100 mg. Diphenhydramine is now available over-the-counter in 25 mg forms. The drug is anticholinergic and can be used for acute dystonic reactions to antipsychotics (see Chapter 4). Promethazine (Phenergan) is a phenothiazine without antipsychotic properties that is marketed as an antihistamine with sedative properties. Again, it is occasionally found useful as a mild sedative at doses of 25-100 mg, but is not a major psychiatric drug. Pyrilamine maleate, another antihistamine, is the ingredient that is used in most over-the-counter preparations (e.g., Compoz) that are used for either tranquilization or hypnosis.

Table 7-C. Other Nighttime Hypnotic Agents

Generic Name	Brand Name	Dosage Forms	Dosage (mg)*
chloral hydrate	Noctec	Capsules: 250/500 mg Concentrate: 500 mg/ml (16 oz bottles)	500–1500
ethchlorvynol	Placidyl	Capsules: 100/200/ 500/750 mg	500–750
ethinamate	Valmid	Capsules: 500 mg	500–1000
glutethimide	Doriden	Tablets: 250/500 mg	250–500
methyprylon	Noludar	Tablets: 50/200 mg Capsules: 300 mg	200–400 300

* Adult dosages. Patients may require slightly higher dosages of chloral hydrate or ethchlorvynol. For child dosages, consult *PDR* or similar reference.

"NONBARBITURATE" HYPNOTICS

In the late 1940s and 1950s several nonbarbiturate hypnotic drugs were developed in the hope that they would be safer and better than the barbiturates. Unfortunately, this hope was not realized. They proved, generally, to have as many limitations as the barbiturates. Only one of these currently available for use is generally viewed as safe and effective. This is chloral hydrate, which in doses between 500 and 1500 mg at bedtime is a somewhat effective and reasonably safe sleeping medication (Table 7-C and Figure 7-2). Early prescription practices of 500 mg at sleep often proved inadequate to produce sedation, and most prescribers have come to favor 1000 mg particularly in younger adult patients. The drug is often used in double-blind trials of other psychiatric medications as an adjunct medication because of its presumed safety and "cleanliness." It is hard to tell whether this reputation is fully deserved, particularly since chloral hydrate itself was once widely abused in England in the early 1900s.

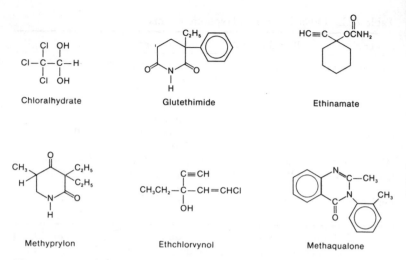

Figure 7-2. Chemical Structures of Nonbarbiturate Hypnotics

Another hypnotic, paraldehyde, is a colorless liquid with a very pungent odor and a burning disagreeable taste. The oral hypnotic dose is 5 or 10 ml. However, the medication has no advantages and may be quite toxic if the material is old and deteriorated. It is too irritating to be given parenterally. Paraldehyde's old place in the detoxification of chronic alcoholics is now supplanted by longer acting and safer benzodiazepines.

Other "nonbarbiturate" hypnotics, including glutethimide, ethinamate, methyprylon, and ethchlorvynol, were developed because of the known dangers of addiction and lethality on suicidal ingestion of the barbiturates (Figure 7-2). Unfortunately, none of these drugs proved to be either safer or less capable of producing physical or psychic dependence than the drugs which they were supposed to replace. There are presently no logical reasons for using them in preference to the safer benzodiazepines. (For further information see Table 7-C.)

METHAQUALONE

Methaqualone (Quaalude) deserves some passing mention (Figure 7-2). This is the most recent of the nonbarbiturate hypnotics marketed as a safe and effective replacement for the more dangerous older sleeping pills. It became widely abused in the illicit street market and achieved a good deal of publicity as the "love" drug in the 1960s. Methaqualone was alleged to have aphrodisiac properties, a proposition which has never been specifically tested in any scientific way. The drug, however, can cause paresthesia, which may somehow increase sexual feelings. It has acquired a remarkably tainted reputation and is now no longer available for prescription use. Whether or not the drug is really more likely to be abused or more euphoriant than the barbiturates is quite unclear. The one available study relevant to the point suggests that it is really no different from pentobarbital in its subjective effects. In our local clinical experience over the past few years we have found occasional patients with severe insomnia who claim methaqualone is far superior as a hypnotic—both in terms of speed of onset and lack of hangover—than other available hypnotics, even comparable barbiturates. In any event, methaqualone, for good or for bad, is no longer available.

L-TRYPTOPHAN

A hypnotic drug that seems to be really free from dependence or abuse liability is the amino acid L-tryptophan. It has not been formally approved for medical use as a hypnotic drug in the United States but is available in both drug stores and health food stores as a dietary supplement either in the pure form or combined with other nutriments. There is reasonable evidence that, at doses of 1-6 g at bedtime, L-tryptophan has some efficacy as a sleeping pill in some patients with insomnia. It is neither as powerful as the major hypnotics nor, presumably, as dangerous. It is, however, a rather expensive way to get a night's sleep, since the drug costs almost $1.00 per g under most circumstances.

Starting dose should be 1-2 g at bedtime with an increase to 3-4 g after two to three nights. The amount of available L-tryptophan in milk—particularly when warmed—rivals a 2 g dose, and some clinicians have advocated this time-honored approach for insomnia. Some workers have further noted that carbohydrates facilitate the absorption of L-tryptophan, suggesting that milk and cookies may be better than milk alone. We know of no double-blind studies of this, however.

Bibliography

Chen C-N: Sleep, depression and antidepressants. Br J Psychiatry 135:385–402, 1970

Dement W, Seidel W, Carskadon M, et al: Changes in daytime sleepiness/alertness with nighttime benzodiazepines, in Pharmacology of Benzodiazepines. Edited by Usdin E, Skolnick P, Tallman JF, et al. New York, Macmillan, 1982, pp 219–228

Falco M: Methaqualone misuse: Foreign experience and US drug control policy. Int J Addict 11:597–610, 1976

Gillin JC, Reynolds CF, Shipley JE: Sleep studies in selected adult neuropsychiatric disorders, in Psychiatry Update, vol 4. Edited by Hales RE, Frances AJ. Washington, DC, American Psychiatric Press, 1985

Greenblatt DJ, Shader RI, Abernethy DR: Current status of benzodiazepines [first of two parts]. N Engl J Med 309:354–359, 1983

Greenblatt DJ, Shader RI, Abernethy DR: Current status of benzodiazepines [second of two parts]. N Engl J Med 309:410–415, 1983

Jasinski D, Griffith J, Prenick J, et al: Unpublished progress report from the Clinical Pharmacology Section of the NIDA Addiction Research Center, Proceedings of the 39th Annual Scientific Meeting, Committee on Problems of Drug Dependence, 1977, pp 133–168

Kales A: Benzodiazepines in the treatment of insomnia, in Pharmacology of Benzodiazepines. Edited by Usdin E, Skolnick P, Tallman JF, et al. New York, Macmillan, 1982, pp 199–217

Roffwarg H, Erman M: Evaluation and diagnosis of the sleep disorders: implications for psychiatry and other clinical specialties, in Psychiatry Update, vol 4. Edited by Hales RE, Frances AJ. Washington, DC, American Psychiatric Press, 1985, pp 294–328

Seidel WF, Roth T, Roehrs T, et al: Treatment of a 12 hour shift of sleep schedule with benzodiazepines. Science 224:1262–1264, 1985

Stimulants

The main available stimulant drugs with some evidence for utility in psychiatric conditions are d-amphetamine, methylphenidate, and magnesium pemoline, although a number of other amphetamine-like substances are marketed for use in weight reduction (Table 8-A). In addition, one interesting anorexiant, fenfluramine, is not a stimulant and probably does not deserve to be classified as an amphetamine but may have some minor uses in psychiatric conditions (e.g., infantile autism).

Amphetamine, originally available as a racemic amphetamine preparation, was in fact the first nonbarbiturate drug to be clinically effective in modern psychopharmacology. It was developed in the late 1930s and studied in children with severe behavior disorders, a condition originally called hyperactivity or minimal brain dysfunction, and more recently and more accurately classified under *DSM-III* as Attentional Deficit Disorder. In this condition all three drugs—d-amphetamine, methylphenidate, and magnesium pemoline—are clearly more effective than placebo. The dose for d-amphet-

8

Table 8-A. Stimulants

Generic Name	Brand Name	Preparations
d-amphetamine	Dexedrine	Tablets: 5 mg Spansules: 5/10/15 mg Elixir: 5 mg/5 ml (16 oz bottles)
methylphenidate	Ritalin	Tablets: 5/10/20 mg Slow Release Tablets: 20 mg
magnesium pemoline	Cylert	Tablets: 18.75/37.5/75 mg

amine is 5-40 mg a day, for methylphenidate 10-80 mg a day, and for magnesium pemoline 18.75-150 mg per day.

All three drugs probably act by releasing dopamine into the synapse and may or may not also have direct agonist activity. They also have noradrenergic actions. In laboratory animals they increase motor activity and at very high doses produce repetitive "compulsive" behavior, including sniffing, staring and paw-chewing. All three drugs tend to increase pulse rate and to a lesser extent blood pressure in high doses, and they tend to decrease appetite and to interfere with sleep. d-Amphetamine and methylphenidate, but not magnesium pemoline, are self-administered intravenously by laboratory animals and are well known to have abuse liability in humans. The major abuse of stimulants has been in the form of methamphetamine, which was used intravenously in very high doses during the flower-child period of the 1960s, resulting in heavily dependent individuals known as "speed freaks." Such individuals usually took the medication in relatively large doses in runs of a few days and then crashed for a day or two before starting up again. Earlier patterns of oral abuse were less intense and dramatic.

There is reasonable evidence that very high doses of d-amphetamine, generally over 80 mg a day and sometimes as high as 1000-2000 mg a day, can produce an acute psychosis which generally resembles paranoid schizophrenia but can occasionally present with delirium and other conventional signs of toxic drug psychosis. This condition is sometimes considered a model for schizophrenia or at least for acute paranoid psychosis.

Of the three drugs, magnesium pemoline is a little different in having a somewhat slower onset and offset of action, making it preferred in occasional patients who get symptom relief for three or four hours from a single dose of methyl-phenidate or *d*-amphetamine with an abrupt change in status as the drug wears off. In such patients magnesium pemoline may be smoother and better tolerated. Child psychiatrists are concerned about hepatocellular damage due to magnesium pemoline and recommend a monthly check of liver function (see Chapter 12). We have not yet run into such a problem in adult patients. The ability of magnesium pemoline prescriptions to be refilled and phoned into the pharmacies makes it the most flexible stimulant to use clinically.

USES OF STIMULANTS

Attentional Deficit Disorder

This is the only condition other than narcolepsy and weight reduction for which stimulants are approved currently by the Food and Drug Administration. In children, the syndrome is manifested by very short attention span, overactivity, irritability, poor social relations, impulsivity, occasional angry or assaultive behavior, poor school performance, and apparent inability to benefit from instruction or limit-setting. Some children with the syndrome have a parent with a history of or current symptoms of a similar condition. Occasional children with the syndrome have clear evidence of central nervous system damage at birth or subsequently; the majority of such patients, however, do not have any clear evidence of "hard" neurological signs of clearly diagnosable brain injury or abnormality.

In children with attentional deficit disorder, any of the three drugs are likely to be clinically better than placebo in about 70-80 percent of those treated; about 30 percent show a clear and highly impressive degree of clinical improvement, and another 40 percent show some modulation of behavior which may be of some clinical importance. Occasionally, children are made more active by the drug. In the first weeks of treatment children often look drawn and even somewhat depressed and rarely show any euphoriant effect from the medication. It is not clear that the drugs dramatically reduce activity level but probably act by improving attention span and organizing behavior more effectively. Some degree of growth inhibition or weight loss has been reported in children but is not a large or general problem.

Wender et al. (1985) at the University of Utah, Huessey (1979) at the University of Vermont, and others have identified adults with symptoms resembling those seen in children with attentional deficit disorder and have shown that such adults may respond to stimulant therapy. These drug responders are very likely to have been remembered as "hyperkinetic" children by their parents. Some individuals who have had clear clinical benefit from stimulants in childhood continue to require and to benefit from stimulant medication well into adult life. Many children with attentional deficit disorder seem to grow out of the major manifestations of the illness some time in adolescence, although they are often left with residual symptoms of impaired concentration or coping ability which might or might not be benefitted by further stimulant administration.

The interesting and clinically useful aspect of stimulant therapy in either children or adults with attentional deficit disorder is that clinical effects are often clear and dramatic within a day or two of reaching the appropriate dosage. This stands in dramatic contrast to the more conventional antidepressants and antipsychotics, which often take days or even weeks to achieve a satisfactory clinical result.

In clinical practice adults with personality disorder, short attention span, restlessness, hyperactivity, irritability, impulsivity, and related symptoms sometimes present with a history of illicit drug abuse. In such individuals, a trial of a stimulant raises an ethical problem: when it is clear that any stimulant will be abused, the drug cannot be used. Stimulants can be used in patients with a history of drug abuse under the following circumstances:

1. When the stimulant drug has clearly been used to improve functioning rather than to produce euphoria or to get "high";
2. When a good therapeutic alliance is available;
3. When the medication can be closely monitored, perhaps in an inpatient setting;
4. When other approaches have failed; and
5. When the patient's problems are seriously interfering with his or her life functioning.

Some children and adults with attentional deficit disorder respond to desipramine, and this can be used in patients who might abuse a stimulant.

Depression

In the early literature on the use of amphetamine in psychiatry, there were a number of case reports of individuals presenting with the full syndrome of endogenous depression who responded dramatically to racemic amphetamine. There have been a few double-blind trials completed at one time or another over the past 30 years which show some evidence of clinical efficacy of stimulants in depressed outpatients. Not all studies are positive; some are only weakly positive and some are clearly negative.

Given the bad repute into which stimulants have fallen, it is probably not reasonable to conduct further trials of

noted. Positive effects—clearing of confusion—occur rapidly, within 10-15 minutes.

Physostigmine may produce intense nausea and vomiting either because of central or peripheral effects. Seizures have also been reported. For these reasons, repeated administrations of physostigmine—outside of an intensive care setting—are not recommended. At one time, some investigators advocated using physostigmine in combination with methscopolamine; however, this combination did not always block the emetic effects of the physostigmine, probably because they represent both central and peripheral effects.

MAOIs in Combination with TCAs

One of the most controversial of combinations is MAOIs with TCAs. Although proscribed in *PDR*, the combination can be relatively safe and is occasionally effective in patients who have failed to respond to treatment with an MAOI or TCA alone. As indicated in Chapter 3, MAOIs when prescribed with sympathomimetic agents can result in acute hypertensive crises. Since TCAs exert an effect on sympathetic systems, prudence is warranted. Early fears of the combination came largely from a number of deaths that resulted from overdosages of the combination. However, overdosages of either TCAs or MAOIs alone can be lethal.

In contrast to these reports, some clinicians have argued that the combination can be of unique benefit. However, double-blind studies comparing a TCA, an MAOI, and the combination in non-treatment-resistant depressed patients have in recent years failed to show the combination is of added benefit. However, the combination also does not appear to be more dangerous. Indeed, recent studies in humans and in animals suggest that some tricyclics may protect against hypertensive crises although they may not afford protection against hyperpyrexic reactions.

The lack of superior efficacy for the MAOI-TCA combi-

stimulants in fresh non-treatment-resistant depressed patients. However, in patients with chronic treatment-resistant depression which has failed to respond to a range of standard antidepressants, stimulants will occasionally provide excellent symptomatic relief and will enable the patient to function adequately for prolonged periods without side effects and without any indication that the drug is being abused or misused. Some of these patients have clear endogenous symptoms, others appear to have atypical depressions of one sort or another, and still others have major symptoms of fatigue or neurasthenia. It is not possible to tell in advance which depressed patients will benefit, although Rickels et al. (1970) suggest that relatively heavy intake of coffee (four cups a day or more) is a predictor of clinical response, at least to magnesium pemoline.

Stimulants also have a place in the crisis management of individuals whose functioning is impaired by depression and whose life situation will deteriorate rapidly if they are not able to resume functioning within a few days. In such situations a trial of methylphenidate or d-amphetamine or magnesium pemoline is worth initiating to attempt to get a patient through a crisis period where failure to function might result in his being fired from his job or being flunked out of college.

In such situations one may well begin with magnesium pemoline because it is the least abusable of the stimulants and also because it can be prescribed by telephone and prescriptions can be refilled, options not available with d-amphetamine or methylphenidate, which are Class II drugs. A good initial dose is 37.5 mg to be given in the morning with a repeat dose in the early afternoon if the initial dose is helpful. If the dose is overstimulating, half a tablet (18.75 mg) can be tried instead. If the dose has no appreciable effect, it can be doubled or even tripled in the morning and again later in the day as needed, up to 75 mg twice a day. Usually within a few days it is clear whether the patient has had a distinct improvement in mental status and functioning. Patients should be advised that if the drug is unpleasantly stimulating or produces any undesirable side effects, they should stop taking it at once and contact their physician. If magnesium pemoline is ineffective or if the patient finds it either sedative or oddly dysphoric, then methylphenidate or *d*-amphetamine may work instead. With these drugs, doses up to 20 or 30 mg of *d*-amphetamine a day or twice that amount of methylphenidate can be tried.

Some patients will show an initial excellent response to a stimulant medication and then develop rapid tolerance and lose all effect, while others will go on and continue to benefit from the same low dose of the stimulant for months or even years. Other patients feel anxious, agitated, and unpleasantly "wired" on all stimulants. If the drug is to be stopped, it can be either tapered or stopped abruptly. Some rebound depression may occur (see Chapter 11).

d-Amphetamine is available in 10 mg or 15 mg spansule (slow release) formulations. Some patients respond better to titrating their dose with tablets while others do better on the spansule.

Phenylpropanolamine is marketed as an over-the-counter antiobesity pill in 37.5 mg and 75 mg dosage strengths, usually in a sustained release preparation. We have seen occasional patients with either depression or attentional deficit disorder who have found phenylpropanolamine helpful in the way a standard stimulant sometimes is. However, most patients and most recreational drug users find the subjective effects of phenylpropanolamine mildly unpleasant. When phenylpropanolamine was abused in "triple threat" illicit pills containing ephedrine and caffeine as well, it is likely that the ephedrine or the combination accounted for the pills' amphetamine-like properties. Phenylpropanolamine alone may reduce appetite and increase pulse and blood pressure a little but is not a useful stimulant. It should be noted that the drug marketed in Europe as phenylpropanolamine is, in fact, a different stereoisomer and does have amphetamine-like stimulant effects.

Drug Combinations. Methylphenidate and *d*-amphetamine both interact with imipramine in laboratory animals to potentiate response to electrical stimulation of pleasure centers. Part of this is pharmacokinetic in the sense that the stimulant and the tricyclic interfere with each other's metabolism causing higher blood levels of each. This property is sometimes used clinically when methylphenidate is prescribed early in tricyclic therapy to hasten response. If a patient improves on methylphenidate plus imipramine it is impossible to tell for sure whether the clinical response is due to a) the methylphenidate alone, b) a longer period on imipramine, c) the elevation of imipramine blood level caused by methylphenidate, or d) a true combined effect of the two drugs. Generally we do not recommend this approach.

Intuitively, it should be considered clinically dangerous to combine a stimulant with an MAOI, since the addition of a stimulant *could* precipitate a hypertensive crisis. However, we know a few patients who have, on their own responsibility, added magnesium pemoline, methylphenidate, *d*-amphetamine, or cocaine to reverse MAOI-induced sedation or lack of clinical response, with alleged good subjective effects and no apparent effect on blood pressure. Other such patients were recently described in the literature. We have seen hypertensive crises when phenylpropanolamine was added to an MAOI, but so far we have not encountered any on stimulant-MAOI combinations. Stimulant-MAOI combinations are not recommended in general practice because the exact degree of risk is not known (see Chapter 3).

Psychosis

Although the older literature from the 1930s and 1940s on the use of racemic amphetamine, *d*-amphetamine, and methylphenidate in patients with then- called chronic schizophrenia is mixed (some patients improved on stimulant given alone, some showed no change, and some worsened), more recent studies of single doses of intravenous methylphenidate show that it increases psychosis in acutely ill patients with manic or schizophrenic disorders but has only a mild stimulant effect when such patients are in remission. More recently, studies by Angrist et al. (1980) and Lieberman et al. (1983) show that chronically ill schizophrenic outpatients who show increased psychosis after a single dose of a stimulant are much more likely to relapse into a psychotic exacerbation than are patients who show no worsening on stimulant administration.

Another drug, fenfluramine, chemically resembles amphetamine but pharmacologically has serotonergic rather than dopaminergic effects. It is available clinically for use in obesity and is generally sedative rather than stimulant. On the basis of local experience in a few patients, fenfluramine raises tricyclic blood levels substantially when given in 20-40 mg a day doses to patients who run very low tricyclic blood levels despite adequate oral doses (e.g., 300 mg of imipramine). We have tried adding fenfluramine to the drug regimen of psychiatric patients gaining excess weight on a variety of classes of drug in the hope that fenfluramine would promote weight reduction without aggravating psychosis or mania (fenfluramine was once studied in mania and had weak antimanic effects). Unfortunately, fenfluramine has, so far, not fulfilled its theoretical promise as a "safe" anorexiant in psychiatric patients. It is safe but does not cause weight loss.

A series of recent papers, published and unpublished, have dealt with the use of fenfluramine in autism. The drug lowers blood serotonin levels, which are sometimes elevated in autism. So far the evidence suggests that some autistic patients function better on fenfluramine, those with higher IQs responding better. The original idea that patients with the higher blood serotonin levels respond best appears to be incorrect, but there is some relation between the observed decrease in blood serotonin and response. There is a suggestion, however, that long-term fenfluramine exposure may cause neurotoxicity in laboratory animals. This new research area has been reviewed by Biederman (1985).

Use Versus Abuse

We occasionally have seen patients who have, in the past, taken prescribed stimulants for years with claimed excellent relief of depression, fatigue, or disorganized behavior and have been taken off the drug by a physician concerned about "drug abuse." Such patients often have then failed to respond to a variety of more conventional tricyclic antidepressants and have been dysphoric and unable to function adequately for years. When the stimulant is represcribed, these patients often do quite well again for prolonged periods. It may be very hard to tell whether such individuals (who rarely have histories suggestive of attention deficit disorder) really have a uniquely stimulant-responsive disorder or whether they somehow have become "dependent" on stimulants. Either way, if they cope well and feel well only on stimulants, take low to moderate dosages as prescribed, and do not develop tolerance, the stimulant should be continued. If the physician feels uncomfortable about prescribing stimulants in such patients, consultation with a clinical psychopharmacologist may provide helpful clinical and ethical support.

More difficult permutations of the problem exist, of course. What about a patient who recalls d-amphetamine as making him feel "better" but not better enough to actually complete graduate courses or even to motivate him to pay the bill of the psychiatrist who was prescribing the pills? What about a patient who has failed on several tricyclics but refuses to try an MAOI because of the restricted diet and risks? Should he be forced to fail on an MAOI before a stimulant is tried or retried? What about a marginally employed, vague, mildly paranoid young man with severe ear pain of an undiagnosable nature who buys illicit stimulants to relieve the pain? The stimulants do not help him function, they do not make him more paranoid—they only make him feel better. What about the chronically very depressed woman who only feels better on 200 mg of methylphenidate a day?

We feel more comfortable prescribing stimulants when they either obviously improve functioning or when they at least relieve incapacitating distress, and we would not force a patient to try an MAOI if he has already improved on a stimulant in the past, but these are personal judgments.

In summary, we suspect that the useful, rapidly acting stimulant drugs are underutilized in American psychiatry—they do not always work or even help, but when they do they can be very effective. It is too early to tell whether bupropion, which resembles the stimulants in some respects (see Chapter 3), will provide a safer, less abusable drug that will help those psychiatric patients who now only respond to standard stimulants.

Bibliography

Angrist B, Peselow E, Rubinstein M, et al: Amphetamine response and relapse risk after depot neuroleptic discontinuation. Psychopharmacology 85:277–283, 1985

Angrist B, Rotrosen J, Gershon S: Responses to apomorphine, amphetamine, and neuroleptics in schizophrenic subjects. Psychopharmacology 67:31–38, 1980

August GJ, Naftali R, Papanicolaou AC, et al: Fenfluramine treatment in infantile autism: neurochemical electrophysiological and behavioral effects. J Nerv Ment Dis 172:604–612, 1984

Biederman G: Fenfluramine (Pondimin) in autism. Biological Therapies in Psychiatry 8:25–28, 1985

Cole JO: Drug therapy of adult minimal brain dysfunction, in Psychopharmacology Update. Edited by Cole JO. Lexington, Mass, Collamore Press, 1981, pp 69–80

Cole JO (ed): The amphetamines in psychiatry. Seminars in Psychiatry 1:128–137, 1969

Davidoff E, Reifenstein E: Treatment of schizophrenia with sympathomimetic drugs: benzedrine sulfate. Psychiatr Q 13:127–144, 1939

Elizur A, Wintner I, Davidson S: The clinical and psychological effects of pemoline in depressed patients—a controlled study. International Pharmacopsychiatry 14:127–134, 1979

Ellinwood EH: Amphetamine psychosis: individuals, settings, and sequences, in Current Concepts on Amphetamine Abuse [DHEW publication no HSM 729085]. Edited by Ellinwood EH, Cohen S. Washington, DC, US Government Printing Office, pp 143–158

Feighner JP, Herbstein J, Damlouji N: Combined MAOI, TCA, and direct stimulant therapy of treatment-resistant depression. J Clin Psychiatry 46:206–209, 1985

Huessey H: Clinical explorations in adult MBD, in Psychiatric Aspects of Minimal Brain Dysfunction in Adults. Edited by Bellak L. New York, Grune and Stratton, 1979

Kaufmann M, Murray G, Cassem N: Use of psychostimulants in medically ill depressed patients. Psychosomatics 23:817–819, 1982

Lieberman J, Kane J, Gadaletta D, et al: The use of methylphenidate challenge test as a predictor of relapse in schizophrenia. Paper presented at American Psychiatric Association Meeting, New York, May 5, 1983

Myerson A: The effect of benzedrine sulfate on mood and fatigue in normal and neurotic persons. AMA Archives of Neurology and Psychiatry 36:816–822, 1936

Rickels K, Gordon P, Gansman D, et al: Pemoline and methylphenidate in mildly depressed outpatients. Clin Pharmacol Ther 11:698–710, 1970

Ritvo ER, Freeman BJ, Yuwiler A: Study of fenfluramine in outpatients with the syndrome of autism. J Pediatr 105:823–828, 1984

Wender PH, Reimherr FW, Wood D, et al: A controlled study of methylphenidate in the treatment of attention deficit disorder, residual type in adults. Am J Psychiatry 142:547–552, 1985

Wood DR, Reinherr FW, Wender PH, et al: Diagnosis and treatment of minimal brain dysfunction in adults: a preliminary report. Arch Gen Psychiatry 33:1453–1460, 1976

Combination and Adjunctive Treatments

It is the general hope of all clinicians that patients will respond to a single psychotherapeutic agent. However, this is usually the exception rather than the rule. Although there has been much warranted consternation regarding polypharmacy (patients receiving too many different types of medications), some patients do require simultaneous treatment with different classes of drugs. Until more is learned about the biochemistry of various disorders and the range of pharmacologic effects of available and future medications, clinicians will constantly be faced with using more than one agent to effect a positive response in individual patients. Obviously, the number of potential combinations is vast and beyond the scope of this chapter. We recommend that clinicians become familiar with a number of commonly used combination drugs or combination regimens that have been reported in recent years to be particularly effective in specific clinical situations. In addition, clinicians should become familiar with combinations that can pose potential difficulties because of drug/drug interactions or additive side effects.

9

Table 9-A.   Combination Antidepressants

Generic Name	Brand Name	Dosage Forms*	Dosage Schedule (mg)†
chlordiazepoxide and amitriptyline	Limbitrol	Tablets: 5–12.5/ 10–25 mg	To start: 3–4/ day of 10–25 mg tabs then 2–6/ day as needed
perphenazine and amitriptyline	Etrafon	Tablets: 2–10/ 2–24/4–10/ 4–25 mg	To start: 1 2–25 or 4–25 TID or QID up to 8/day of any strength
	Triavil	Tablets: 2–10/ 2–25/4–10/ 4–25/4–50 mg	To start: 1 2–25 or 4–25 TID or QID or 1 4–50 with increases to a maximum of 4 4–50/day or 8/day of other strengths

* Dosage forms list amount (mg) of first and second ingredients, respectively.
† Adult dosages. Some patients may require lower doses.

(The use of antiparkinsonians and benzodiazepines in combination with neuroleptics is discussed in detail in Chapter 4; other possible combinations are discussed throughout the text.)

AMITRIPTYLINE-PERPHENAZINE

Amitriptyline, a tricyclic antidepressant, is marketed in combination with a phenothiazine antipsychotic—perphenazine. This combination appears under two trade names: Triavil and Etrafon (Table 9-A). Various combinations of strengths are available, and these are coded according to the dose of each drug contained in the capsule; the dosage of perphenazine is given first. For example, a capsule of Triavil or Etrafon 2-25 contains 2 mg of perphenazine and 25 mg of amitriptyline (Table 9-A). This neuroleptic-tricyclic combination is widely used in the United States, generally prescribed by primary care practitioners. However, experienced psycho-pharmacologists advocate prescribing these drugs individually to allow for optimum flexibility in dosing.

The indications for this combination are anxiety and agitation associated with depression in both neurotic and psychotic patients, including schizophrenia, as well as physical disease. Theoretically and practically, these agents might best be used to treat patients with psychotic depression, an illness that often responds more favorably to this combination or electroconvulsive therapy than to tricyclics alone. This preferential response suggests a possible involvement of dopaminergic systems in delusional depression.

One major issue that has arisen is whether the combination's preferential benefit in delusional depression is really due to its combined pharmacologic effects rather than to the higher blood levels of amitriptyline produced by simultaneously prescribing a phenothiazine (see the section on Tricyclic Blood Levels in Chapter 3). Data from double-blind studies of Spiker et al. (1981) comparing perphenazine, amitriptyline, and the combination in delusional depression suggest that the additive pharmacologic properties of the combination are of paramount importance rather than the enhanced tricyclic blood levels. However, the relatively higher TCA plasma levels attained with such combination drugs could help explain the early studies in nondeluded depressed patients that showed reasonable antidepressant efficacy using combinations that contained relatively low doses of the tricyclic. Conceivably, in those early studies, patients responded because they were attaining relatively higher TCA plasma levels than they would if prescribed a TCA alone.

Perphenazine-amitriptyline will produce greater anticholinergic effects than amitriptyline alone because of increased plasma levels as well as additive anticholinergic effects. Fortunately, perphenazine produces relatively limited anticholinergic side reactions, making this less of an issue than for other potential combinations of phenothiazines and amitriptyline. For example, thioridazine produces the most pronounced anticholinergic side effects and when added to amitriptyline—the most potent anticholinergic of the tricyclics—can result in marked anticholinergic reactions. This combination should obviously be used with caution.

The recommended starting dose of Triavil is one 2-25 or 4-25 tablet three times per day or two 4-50 tablets per day. The maintenance dose is two to four tablets per day. For elderly and adolescent patients, the recommended starting dose is one 4-10 Triavil tablet three times per day. We recommend that clinicians opt for prescribing the components of amitriptyline-perphenazine compounds individually to allow for increased flexibility. This is particularly important so as to avoid extended exposure to phenothiazine. Long-term use of phenothiazines can result in tardive dyskinesia, which has been reported as possibly being more common in patients with major affective disorders than in those with schizophrenia (see Chapter 4).

AMITRIPTYLINE-CHLORDIAZEPOXIDE

The combination of amitriptyline and chlordiazepoxide was introduced into the United States in 1980 and marketed under the brand name of Limbitrol (Table 9-A). It carries an FDA-approved indication for the treatment of patients with mixed anxiety-depression. The numerical designation parallels that of Triavil. (Limbitrol 10-25 contains 10 mg of chlordiazepoxide and 25 mg of amitriptyline.) It is also available in a 5-12.5 form (Table 9-A). The recommended starting dose in adults is three to four tablets per day of the 10-25 strength with a recommended maximum daily dose of six tablets per day. In elderly patients, the recommended starting dose is one 5-12.5 tablet TID-QID.

Although data from previous studies indicate that chlordiazepoxide alone is not an effective antidepressant, the combination has been shown to decrease anxiety, to aid sleep early in treatment (within the first two weeks), and to be associated with better patient compliance. However, published studies do not indicate that continued benefit can be obtained after the initial four to six weeks. Wherever possible, clinicians who have used the combination for this initial period should consider switching to prescribing these agents individually and eventually tapering the benzodiazepine.

There are considerable differences between combinations of amitriptyline with perphenazine and those with chlordiazepoxide. Enhanced efficacy of the combination early in treatment is not due to any increase in TCA plasma levels, since benzodiazepines, unlike antipsychotics, do not slow microsomal enzymatic activity in the liver. (However, since chlordiazepoxide does not increase TCA plasma levels, six 10-25 tablets per day may produce an inadequate TCA blood level for many seriously depressed patients.) The benzodiazepines are not anticholinergic and do not pose a problem in this regard. They can, however, add to the sedation produced by amitriptyline alone.

L-TRIIODOTHYRONINE-TCA COMBINATIONS

A number of years ago a debate emerged in the literature as to whether thyroid preparations (e.g., L-triiodothyronine [T_3]) when prescribed with a TCA hastened the speed of onset of the antidepressant effect. Early studies in women suggested it did, although later studies in men, which also employed higher dosages of tricyclics, failed to substantiate the early finding. Then, a fallow period followed for this combination until 1982, when Goodwin et al. reported that the addition of 25-50 µg/day of L-triiodothyronine (Cytomel) brought out within seven days a clinical response in patients who had previously not responded to a seemingly adequate TCA trial. A number of subsequent clinical reports have confirmed this observation, although some clinicians have reported responses requiring seven to 10 days of combined therapy. We believe it is reasonable to add 25 μg/day of L-triiodothyronine for seven days to a tricyclic before switching to another antidepressant. This can be further increased to 37.5 μg or 50 μg for an additional week if only a limited change is seen at day seven. Generally, patients experience little additional side effects, although we have occasionally seen patients complain of headaches or of feeling warm. If a patient responds positively, we recommend continuing the L-triiodothyronine for an additional 60 days and then tapering by 12.5 μg every three days. Some patients will demonstrate a resumption of symptoms and will require reinstitution of the L-triiodothyronine. Overall, it is our impression that Cytomel is most useful in patients with pronounced psychomotor retardation. We have on occasion found that it can also bring out a response in patients who have relapsed while on a tricyclic to which they had previously responded.

The mechanism of action of T_3 potentiation of tricyclics is undetermined. Generally, theories have revolved around its facilitating receptor adaptation. However, Targum et al. (1983) reported that T_3 responders had demonstrated relatively enhanced thyroid-stimulating hormone responses to thyrotropin-releasing hormone infusions, suggesting that a subtle form of thyroid dysfunction might play a role in these patients.

LITHIUM-TCA COMBINATIONS

Lithium has been well studied in its own right as an antidepressant. Overall, the drug is effective in some 50 percent of patients, with suggestions that it is best used in males with bipolar depression (see Chapters 3 and 5). de Montigny et al. (1981, 1983) reported that the addition of lithium carbonate to a tricyclic trial resulted in clinical improvement within seven to 14 days in patients who had failed to respond to a TCA alone. These observations have been confirmed in two double-blind studies. Response is often at low dosages

(900-1200 mg/day) and at low serum levels (<0.8 mEq/L). The mechanism of action has been hypothesized as a potentiation of serotonergic activity—either via increased biosynthesis or receptor adaptation. Our experience with the combination has been generally favorable and we have been particularly impressed with results obtained in depressed patients with pronounced obsessionality and agitation. Price et al. (1983) reported that lithium carbonate also elicited a response in patients with delusional depression who had not responded to perphenazine-amitriptyline alone. Overall, we would not expect more than 50 percent of TCA nonresponders to respond to the addition of either L-triiodothyronine (Cytomel) or lithium carbonate. The clinician should strongly consider either one of these strategies before switching to other antidepressants. If lithium carbonate is to be added, it should be initiated at 300 mg twice a day for two days and increased to 900 mg/day for three to four days with a further increase to 1200 mg/day for a total 10-14 day trial.

METHYLPHENIDATE-TCA COMBINATIONS

In the early 1970s, Wharton and colleagues reported that the addition of methylphenidate increased plasma levels of tricyclics by inhibiting microsomal degradation of the TCA in the liver (similar to that observed with antipsychotic agents). This approach offers a possible way of increasing TCA plasma levels without increasing the dose of the TCA. In addition to this effect, methylphenidate is a stimulant and may be useful in treating the anergia and psychomotor retardation of endogenous depression. However, as described in the previous chapter, we do not recommend adding methylphenidate for increasing plasma levels, since clinicians can attain higher TCA plasma levels by increasing TCA dosages themselves. Rather, clinicians might want to use methylphenidate for its energizing properties but should keep in mind it may increase TCA plasma levels and side effects.

BETHANECHOL-TCA COMBINATIONS

The anticholinergic effects of the tricyclic antidepressants can be severe (see Chapter 3). Peripherally these include dry mouth, heartburn secondary to esophageal reflux, constipation, urinary hesitance or inability to void, and blurred vision. Central nervous system effects include problems with memory, speech blockage, confusion, and visual hallucinosis.

Peripheral anticholinergic effects may be ameliorated via the introduction of bethanechol (Urecholine)—a cholinergic agonist—in doses ranging between 50 and 150 mg/day. It is usually given as 25 mg TID or QID, increasing the dose to 50 mg TID or QID if neither improvement nor cholinergic side effects (e.g., abdominal cramps) occur; side effects are uncommon. Originally reported in an open study by Everett in 1976, its use, to our knowledge, has not been assessed under double-blind conditions. Our experience has been that bethanechol is more helpful for urinary hesitance than for constipation and blurred vision but that overall it is of limited efficacy. Recently, the acute use of bethanechol to aid patients who develop impotence on TCAs has been advocated; 25 mg is taken an hour or so before attempting intercourse. Here, also, our limited experience has not been particularly favorable.

PHYSOSTIGMINE AS AN ANTICHOLINERGIC ANTIDOTE

When patients develop confusion on TCAs, antiparkinsonian agents, and antipsychotics, clinicians should consider anticholinergic delirium, a major problem when it occurs. This should be managed primarily with dose reduction. The parenteral administration of physostigmine—a cholinesterase inhibitor that crosses the blood-brain barrier—can be used as a possible clinical test for anticholinergic delirium. The drug can be administered in a single 0.5 cc (1.0 mg/cc) dose and may be repeated once after 20-30 minutes if no effect is

nation could reflect the limited dosages of both drugs used—e.g., 45 mg of phenelzine and 150 mg of amitriptyline. Some investigators have reported to us that combining higher dosages of both is effective, and we have noted positive results in some patients. However, generally speaking, a number of important caveats should be noted: 1) It appears safest to start the two drugs together. Adding a TCA to the MAOI is far more dangerous than adding the MAOI to the TCA. 2) Clomipramine when combined with an MAOI (particularly tranylcypromine) is far more likely to produce hypertensive crises and other reactions than are other TCAs. 3) Amitriptyline and trimipramine are believed to be the TCAs that "mix best" with an MAOI, i.e., produce less in the way of hypertensive crises. This is largely unproven although suggestive data do exist. 4) Phenelzine and isocarboxazid appear less problematic than does tranylcypromine, which may have an amphetamine-like action.

Tricyclic-Sedative Hypnotics

Not infrequently, depressed patients will require the addition of a sedative hypnotic to an antidepressant agent. In the case of tricyclics, it is most prudent to use a benzodiazepine, since it will not alter the pharmacokinetics of the antidepressant. Barbiturates and to some extent chloral hydrate will induce microsomal breakdown of tricyclics in the liver, resulting in lower TCA plasma levels. The prolonged use of these drugs should thus be avoided in combination with TCAs whenever possible. Obviously the use of any hypnotic with another psychotropic also requires watching for untoward sedation or central nervous system depression.

Bibliography

de Montigny C, Grunberg F, Mayer A, et al: Lithium induces rapid relief of depression in tricyclic antidepressant drug non-responders. Br J Psychiatry 138:252–255, 1981 de Montigny C, Cournoyer G, Morissette R, et al: Lithium carbonate addition in tricyclic antidepressant-resistant unipolar depression. Arch Gen Psychiatry 40:1327–1334, 1983

Everett HC: The use of bethanecol chloride with tricyclic antidepressants. Am J Psychiatry 132:1202–1206, 1976

Feighner JP, Brauzer B, Gelenberg AJ, et al: A placebo-controlled multicenter trial of limbitrol versus its components (amitriptyline and chlordiazepoxide) in the symptomatic treatment of depressive illness. Psychopharmacology 61:217–225, 1979

Glassman AH, Perel JM: The clinical pharmacology of imipramine. Arch Gen Psychiatry 28:649–653, 1973

Goodwin FK, Prange A, Post R, et al: Potentiation of antidepressant effects by L-triiodothyronine in tricyclic nonresponders. Am J Psychiatry 139:34–38, 1982

Granacher RP, Baldessarini RJ: Physostigmine: its use in acute anticholinergic syndrome with antidepressant and antiparkinson drugs. Arch Gen Psychiatry 23:375–380, 1978

Heninger GR, Charney DS, Sternberg DE: Lithium carbonate augmentation of antidepressant treatment. Arch Gen Psychiatry 40:1335–1342, 1983

Kline NS, Pare M, Hallstrom C, et al: Amitriptyline protects patients on MAOI's from tyramine reactions. J Clin Psychopharmacol 2:434–435, 1982

Pare CMB, Kline N, Hallstrom C, et al: Will amitriptyline prevent the "cheese" reaction of monoamine oxidase inhibitors? Lancet 2:183–186, 1982

Price LH, Conwell Y, Nelson JC: Lithium augmentation of combined neurolelptic-tricyclic treatment in delusional depression. Am J Psychiatry 140:318–322, 1983

Spiker DG, Hanin I, Cofsky J, et al: Pharmacological treatment of delusional depressives. Psychopharmacol Bull 17:201–202, 1981

Targum SD, Greenberg R, Harmon R, et al: Adjunctive thyroid hormone in refractory depression [New Research Abstract 38]. American Psychiatric Association Annual Meeting, New York, May 1983

Wharton RN, Perel JM, Dayton PG, et al: A potential clinical use for methylphenidate with tricyclic antidepressants. Am J Psychiatry 127:1619–1625, 1971

Wheatley D: Potentiation of amitriptyline by thyroid hormone. Arch Gen Psychiatry 26:229–233, 1972

White K, Simpson G: Combined MAOI-tricyclic antidepressant treatment: a reevaluation. J Clin Psychopharmacol 1:264–282, 1981

White K, Razani J, Simpson G, et al: Combined MAOI-tricyclic antidepressant treatment: a controlled trial. Psychopharmacol Bull 18:180–181, 1982

Emergency Room Treatment

Psychiatrists see patients in crisis not only in emergency rooms but also (occasionally) in their offices, during home visits, or in medical or nursing home settings. This chapter deals with problems generally within the scope of the psychiatrist functioning without major laboratory or hospital backup.

In emergency situations, psychiatrists are often faced with the diagnosis and treatment of patients presenting with psychiatric symptoms of sudden or presumed recent onset. Phenomenologically, these can be crudely subdivided into the following:

1. Acute psychotic reactions, usually with overt thought disorder, paranoid ideation, and/or hallucinations, marked fear, or anger;
2. Delirium presenting with disorientation and confusion with or without psychotic symptoms;

10

217

3. Severe anxiety without psychotic symptoms but often with physical symptoms;
4. Anger and belligerent behavior with or without signs of alcohol or other intoxication;
5. Depression with suicidal ideation with or without a recent suicide attempt;
6. Psychogenic stupor.

In some of these situations a history will be obtainable either from the patient or from friends or relatives. In others, the patient may have been carrying enough identification so that friends or relatives can be rapidly contacted. In the worst situation, the psychiatrist will have little to go on besides the patient's behavior and a brief physical examination. When the patient is severely disturbed, obtunded, or confused, can give no history, and has no diagnostic stigmata (e.g., needle tracks, obvious atropine-like toxic signs), hospitalization without specific drug treatment is indicated, or at least medical evaluation with toxic screens, electrocardiogram, etc., in a competent medical emergency facility.

It is necessary to stress the importance of really trying to ascertain which drugs the patient has been taking or may have been taking before beginning pharmacotherapy of psychiatric emergency patients. Deaths have occurred when tricyclic antidepressants or meperidine were given to patients on monoamine oxidase inhibitors. Adding sedative drugs to a patient already intoxicated on alcohol or other sedative drugs is unwise. Adding a neuroleptic to a patient with possible neuroleptic malignant syndrome is obviously contraindicated. Similarly, drugs must be carefully chosen if a tricyclic overdose may have affected cardiac function. In short, it is better to avoid medication if the patient may be on preexisting medication or may have overdosed on an unknown drug until the situation can be clarified.

ACUTE PSYCHOTIC REACTIONS

Psychotic symptoms can be caused by drugs. These should be ruled out by history, physical examination, and urine and/or blood tests for drugs of abuse, wherever possible.

Hallucinogens

Usually LSD or mescaline or related drugs cause visual illusions and distortions of body image, sometimes with panic, grandiose ideas, or suicidal drive, but patients usually have some knowledge of which drug had been ingested. Time and a calm, supportive environment enable most such patients to be "talked down." A sedative drug (e.g., 2 mg of lorazepam, or enough to produce sleep) will give time for the hallucinogen to wear off. Antipsychotics have also been used, but are probably not necessary. There are no characteristic physical stigmata of hallucinogenic intoxication. Very large doses of marijuana or hashish can sometimes produce similar states.

Amphetamines

High doses (over 50 mg) of *d*-amphetamine or equivalent doses of related drugs, including cocaine and phenylpropanolamine, can produce excited, paranoid psychotic states, usually with a clear sensorium but rarely with delirium. Signs of sympathetic overactivity are less common than would be expected. Patients on prolonged high doses of stimulants can show stereotyped behavior such as picking at spots on the skin, lip biting, or tooth grinding. These states tend to respond to dopamine blocking drugs such as haloperidol. The dose required is a function of the degree of excitement, but 5 mg po or im could be used as an initial dose in disturbed but not wildly excited patients. Hospital admission is generally necessary. Amphetamine psychosis can be treated as though it were a real schizophreniform psychosis (see Chapter 4).

Some patients clear in hours or days; others go on to a schizophrenic course of, at best, slow improvement despite adequate medication.

Phencyclidine (PCP)

This drug can not only produce behavior that mimics paranoid schizophrenia or manic states but can also produce even more bizarre, violent behavior than amphetamines or LSD. There is sometimes muscle tension, tachycardia and hypertension, drooling, horizontal and vertical nystagmus, analgesia, or loss of proprioception with ataxia. Because PCP is best excreted only in acid urine, urine tests can be negative while blood tests are positive; both should be done. PCP psychosis is worsened by environmental stimulation. Probably a benzodiazepine (e.g., 1 or 2 mg of lorazepam po or im) is better as emergency medication than a neuroleptic. Patients with severe reactions or symptoms not rapidly abating should be hospitalized.

Anticholinergics

A variety of drugs, including atropine, trihexyphenidyl, and over-the-counter medications containing scopolamine, can induce delirium with psychotic symptoms. Dry, hot, flushed skin, dry mouth, dilated pupils, and tachycardia usually accompany these symptoms. Supportive treatment is indicated, with medical hospitalization.

Physostigmine *will* reverse the symptoms, but only briefly; it can evoke seizures and other adverse effects on its own and should not be used by clinicians who are inexperienced in its use (see Chapter 9).

Alcohol or Sedative Intoxication

Ataxia, slurred speech, confusion, and excitement with belligerent paranoid ideation can be confused with schizophreniform psychosis, but alcohol on the breath or history of sedative ingestion will often clarify the diagnosis. In chronic alcoholics, visual and auditory hallucinosis can complicate the picture.

A differential diagnosis should be made in patients already intoxicated with sedatives to avoid giving additional sedative drugs such as lorazepam or amobarbital.

If tranquilization is needed, an antipsychotic, such as chlorpromazine (25 to 50 mg by mouth) or haloperidol (5 mg parenterally) is a better choice.

Sedative Withdrawal and Delirium Tremens

Delirium with agitation, tremor, disorientation, hallucinosis, confusion, tachycardia, and hypotension occurs in patients undergoing withdrawal from physical dependence on alcohol, barbiturates, or benzodiazepines. In this instance sedative drugs are needed. When in doubt, 25 mg of chlordiazepoxide could be given stat orally. (See Chapter 11 for details of the treatment of sedative dependence.)

Mixed Psychotic Reactions

With any psychotic reaction presumptively due to illicit or licit drug toxicity, a variety of complicated clinical pictures can and do occur. Illicit drug users often take several kinds of drugs and alcohol simultaneously. Schizophrenics abuse drugs and/or become intoxicated on alcohol, and acute drug-induced psychosis can sometimes persist and blend into a picture indistinguishable from schizophrenia which can continue for days or weeks. The pharmacotherapeutic problem is to choose between acute dosages of an antipsychotic versus a benzodiazepine versus watchful waiting while checking for illicit drugs in urine or blood, evaluating possible medical causes, and obtaining a recent history from friends or relatives. A modest oral benzodiazepine dose (e.g., 2 mg of lorazepam,

10 mg of diazepam, or 25 mg of chlordiazepoxide) may be the most conservative option when the diagnosis is in doubt and the patient is very agitated. For parenteral use lorazepam (1 or 2 mg) is more rapidly and reliably absorbed than are the other parenteral benzodiazepines. Benzodiazepines should not be used in patients who appear already intoxicated on alcohol or sedative drugs.

Schizophrenic, Schizophreniform, or Manic Psychosis

When the likelihood of a drug-induced psychosis is low and the patient is manifestly acutely psychotic—paranoid, disorganized, hallucinated, agitated, belligerent, etc.—some experts recommend rapid neuroleptization (e.g., 10 mg of haloperidol im every hour for up to four hours, stopping when the patient becomes calm). There is no real evidence that that much is required. Often oral haloperidol will be taken without objection by the patient; in that case, liquid medication is preferred, since ingestion can be ensured. Whether given by mouth or injection, a single 10 mg dose of haloperidol may well suffice, followed by 5 mg after two hours if the patient is still agitated. Other parenteral anti-psychotics (e.g., 20 mg of thiothixene, 50 mg of chlorpromazine, 25 mg of loxapine) are probably as effective, although chlorpromazine is more sedative and more likely to cause hypotension. An antiparkinsonian drug (e.g., 2 mg of biperiden) should usually be given at the same time as the neuroleptic to help avert dystonia.

In very severe psychotic excitements, 5 mg of droperidol given slowly intravenously will produce sedation and often control excitement within a few minutes. This drug is FDA approved only for "use" in anesthesia but has been used in some psychiatric emergency settings. Lorazepam, 1-2 mg im or iv, will also produce marked sedation on occasion, but intravenous medication should only be used where airways and resuscitation equipment are at hand.

When the psychotic patient can give some history and has a preference among available antipsychotic drugs, or when relatives or past medical records provide relevant information, the "best" past drug for the particular patient should be used.

Delirium

Delirium in medically ill patients seen in emergency rooms should be treated only very cautiously with psychoactive drugs while the underlying medical problem is being diagnosed and treated, preferably after hospital admission.

Severe Anxiety

Patients can present with panic, with severe fear and anxiety, and with multiple somatic symptoms. If medical illness can be rapidly ruled out or the patient has a known history of psychogenic panic atttacks, oral diazepam is probably the treatment of choice because of its rapid onset of action after oral administration and its lack of prolonged sedation. Either 10 mg or 5 mg dosages can be tried, depending on the severity of the anxiety and the patient's past responses to sedatives. Antidepressant drugs are indicated in the longer term treatment of panic disorders but are slow in onset and of no immediate value in a patient experiencing severe anxiety at the time the first dose is given. Diazepam is probably also the drug of choice in anxiety induced by recent severe stress if the stressful situation is now past. One could argue that alprazolam could be preferred in panic disorder patients presenting in panic since the drug can both alleviate the present panic and be continued as a maintenance treatment. It seems better, however, to defer that clinical decision until the acute panic is past (See Chapter 6).

Some experts prefer low dose antipsychotic drugs in patients with borderline or other personality disorders presenting with an acute crisis, but we know of no evidence favoring an antipsychotic over a benzodiazepine in the emergency room situation. If the patient has a past history of sedative abuse, perhaps 25 mg of chlorpromazine could be tried as a sedative antipsychotic *if* the patient is not currently dependent on sedative drugs. If buspirone becomes available for use in anxiety, this non-dependence-inducing antianxiety drug could be used in patients with a history of sedative abuse.

Angry Belligerence

In nonpsychotic patients presenting in emergency rooms with angry tantrums, as well as similar patients with severe anxiety that seems to be based on family fights or other interpersonal crises, supportive listening, reassurance, and the elixir of time will often cause the patient to gradually become calm and reasonable without specific medication. Sedative or alcohol-related angry intoxication will also often pass gradually with time, talk, and external limit setting. If the hostility is severe or persistent, an antipsychotic, perhaps haloperidol (5 mg po or im), can be tried to calm the patient and, hopefully, reduce anger, but no data are available on this use. Benzodiazepine sedatives can sometimes decrease controls and leave the patient more excited and disinhibited.

Depression

Suicidally depressed patients brought to an emergency room after suicide threats or nonharmful attempts present a real challenge to clinical judgment. The conservative course is to admit such patients to a secure inpatient unit. Occasionally, this may seem unwise or impractical. If the clinician can make a relationship with and personally follow the patient—and if friends or relatives can reliably supervise the patient until the next appointment—antidepressant medication can be begun. No antidepressant works fast enough to be dramatically useful in such situations. Trazodone and alprazolam have the advantage of being relatively safe if taken in overdose with suicidal intent. Some clinicians prefer starting the patient on a standard tricyclic, giving the patient only enough pills to last until the next appointment.

Psychogenic Stupor

If medical or neurological causes for stupor can be ruled out, hospital admission to a psychiatric ward is generally indicated. If no information on the patient is available, intravenous sodium amobarbital can sometimes enable a history to be obtained by letting the patient talk relatively freely, but this approach requires a clinician experienced in this technique and, again, is best done in an inpatient setting (See Chapter 6).

Bibliography

Cole J: Drugs and seclusion and restraint. McLean Hospital Journal 10:37–53, 1985

Dubin W, Stolberg R: Emergency psychiatry for the house officer. New York, SP Medical and Scientific Books, 1981

Hyman S (ed): Manual of Psychiatric Emergencies. Boston, Little, Brown, 1984

Shader R (ed): Manual of Psychiatric Therapeutics. Boston, Little, Brown, 1975 [See Chapters 7, 11, 15, and 20]

Pharmacotherapy of Chemical Dependence

Drug therapies for patients with substance use disorders are sometimes necessary or useful but are rarely sufficient to cure the disorder, except in the occasional situation in which illicit drugs are overused by a patient with a major depression to reduce psychic pain or with mania as a manifestation of overactivity and uncontrolled hedonism. In these situations, appropriate drug therapy for the underlying major psychiatric condition *can* be very helpful. Unfortunately, some patients with clear syndromes (e.g., depression, bipolar disorder, or schizophrenia) continue to abuse illicit drugs even when in full or partial remission.

11

There are, however, specific drug therapies for some aspects of chemical dependence. Medications are useful to ameliorate withdrawal symptoms caused by physical dependence on sedative or opiate drugs. Methadone, as maintenance therapy, is a longer acting, more manageable, less dangerous drug than heroin and can be given indefinitely in an attempt to replace heroin. Naltrexone, an opiate antagonist, can also be given indefinitely to prevent the patient from obtaining euphoria from heroin. Disulfiram (Antabuse) is used in chronic alcoholism to ensure that patients will become unpleasantly sick if they consume alcohol.

Some classes of illicit drugs, of course, require no specific drug therapies because they do not cause any serious degree of physical dependence. These include marijuana and the hallucinogens (e.g., LSD, mescaline). Such drugs can be abruptly discontinued, even in the case of heavy and frequent users. Drug dependence syndromes for which drug therapies are sometimes or regularly useful involve stimulants, opiates, sedative-hypnotics, and alcohol.

STIMULANTS

When a patient who is dependent on stimulants is hospitalized, stimulant administration should be stopped abruptly. No tapered withdrawal is necessary.

Patients who have been taking stimulants in large amounts (e.g., over 50 mg of *d*-amphetamine or several doses of cocaine a day) will often have a withdrawal syndrome consisting of depression, fatigue, hyperphagia, and hypersomnia. In unstable individuals this rebound depression could reach serious clinical proportions for a few days and may persist for weeks, usually in less severe form. There have been positive pilot studies of the use of desipramine as a treatment for cocaine or amphetamine abuse. However these limited studies do not provide clearcut guidelines on how to use antidepressants in these patients. It is not entirely clear whether desipramine, given to a patient coming off a stimulant, is serving as a replacement for the abused stimulant or as a treatment for postwithdrawal depression.

The issue of "abuse" is a problem with medically prescribable stimulants. If the patient has a clinical depression which responds uniquely to stimulants or a clear adult attention deficit disorder and takes moderate doses in a stable manner to produce socially responsible functioning, perhaps stimulant use may be therapeutically helpful and worth reconsidering if alternate pharmacotherapies fail. If the patient takes stimulants in large doses to get "high" for euphoriant purposes or pushes dosage to the point that paranoia or other serious symptoms develop, then prescribing stimulants is obviously contraindicated. It is not yet clear whether newer, presumptively dopaminergic antidepressants such as bupropion will be more or less useful than desipramine as a maintenance treatment in stimulant users or abusers (see Chapters 3 and 8).

OPIATES

Detoxification

Abstinence symptoms can begin as early as six hours after the last dose of heroin or other short-acting opiates. Withdrawal symptoms include anxiety, insomnia, yawning, sweating, and rhinorrhea, followed by dilated pupils, tremor, gooseflesh, chills, anorexia, and muscle cramps. About a day after the last dose, pulse, blood pressure, respiration, and temperature may all increase, and diarrhea, nausea, and vomiting can occur. The syndrome, untreated, peaks at two to three days and resolves within about 10 days, although mild variable complaints may persist for weeks.

Because a great deal of street heroin is so weak, some supposed addicts may not have developed true physical dependence. Also both street and medical opiate users with or without real physical dependence often consciously or unconsciously exaggerate their withdrawal distress in an effort to obtain more opiate medication from the physician. For these reasons the drug treatment of the withdrawal syndrome should be based on objective signs of opiate withdrawal, not on subjective complaints. These are listed in Table 11-A.

Methadone, a long-acting opiate, is used to treat with-

Table 11-A.   Objective Opiate Withdrawal Signs

1. Pulse 10 beats per minute or more over baseline or over 90 if no history of tachycardia and baseline unknown (baseline: vital sign values one hour after receiving 10 mg of methadone)
2. Systolic blood pressure 10 mm Hg or more above baseline or over 160/95 in nonhypertensive patients
3. Dilated pupils
4. Gooseflesh, sweating, rhinorrhea, or lacrimation

drawal because of its superior pharmacokinetics (a long half-life). A short-acting drug like morphine would have to be given every few hours to block withdrawal, whereas methadone accomplishes this when given only twice a day.

The initial methadone dose should be 10 mg orally, in liquid or crushed tablet form so as to blind the patient to that dosage and subsequent dosages during detoxification. The patient should be evaluated every four hours, and an additional 10 mg of methadone should be administered if at least two of the four criteria in Table 11-A are met. Unless the patient is being withdrawn from high-dose methadone maintenance therapy, no more than 40 mg of methadone should be required in the first 24 hours.

The total dosage of methadone given in the first 24 hours should be considered the stabilization dose. This dose is then given the next day in two divided doses (e.g., 15 mg at 8:00 A.M. and 8:00 P.M.) in crushed or liquid form and should be consumed under direct observation of a staff member to avoid illicit diversion. The stabilization dose should then be reduced by 5 mg a day until the patient is completely withdrawn.

A patient who is physically dependent on sedative drugs and opiates should be maintained on the stabilization methadone dose without tapering until completely withdrawn from the sedative drug.

An alternative pharmacologic approach to the management of opiate withdrawal has been used for the last few years in some centers. This involves the use of the nonopiate antihypertensive drug, clonidine, which has mixed noradrenergic effects. It can suppress both objective and subjective symptoms of opiate withdrawal. A reasonable initial dose is about 5 µg/kg (0.4 mg for an 80 kg patient). This dose can be given three times a day (e.g., 9:00 A.M., 3:00 P.M., and 9:00 P.M.). The dose is titrated upward or downward depending on the signs and symptoms of opiate withdrawal and clonidine-related side effects. The latter commonly include dry mouth, drowsiness or sedation, constipation, fatigue, dizziness, and headache. In one inpatient study of the use of clonidine in the detoxification of patients coming off maintenance methadone, an average dose of about 1.0 mg of clonidine a day was required for the first eight days off methadone. In a study using clonidine in outpatient detoxification, the medication was begun at 0.1 mg every four to six hours as needed and increased to 0.2 mg every four to six hours with a maximum of 1.2 mg a day (average maximum dose was 0.8 mg). Some variation of these dosing strategies could be used if a methadone detoxification program is to be avoided. Clonidine (Catapres) is available in 0.1, 0.2, and 0.3 mg tablets.

Maintenance

For many years, methadone maintenance has been available in major urban areas in specially licensed clinics as a replacement therapy for heroin or other illicit opiates for confirmed addicts who have failed to stay drug-free after detoxification. The dose adjustment varies from program to program; doses as high as 80 mg a day are used in some clinics. Patients usually take the drug once a day at the clinic under direct supervision and have their urine samples checked for other illicit drug use. If the patient is drug free and doing generally well, "take homes" are often allowed so that the patient only takes the methadone dose at the clinic every other day. The drug is often dispensed in Tang to avoid intravenous misuse of the alternate-day dose taken at home. Although this regimen would seem to provide a popular and useful alternative for confirmed opiate addicts, patients often drop out of methadone maintenance programs after weeks or months of participation.

LAAM (L-alpha-acetyl-methadone) is even longer acting than methadone and would be effective even if administered only three times a week, eliminating the complications of daily clinic visits and the diversion of "take homes." But, despite extensive study, LAAM is not yet approved for prescription use.

Either methadone or LAAM is intended to avert withdrawal symptoms and to abolish craving for opiates in heroin addicts. It is also supposed to provide so high a level of tolerance to opiates that self-administration of street heroin or other illicit morphine-like drugs will no longer elicit euphoria. Maintenance methadone is stabilizing for some opiate addicts but does not completely suppress drug-seeking behavior even for heroin; patients in methadone programs often continue to get in trouble with other drugs of abuse, especially alcohol. Maintenance therapy, even coupled with good support programs, cannot solve the multiple problems of many heroin users. Maintenance methadone is a specialized modality in which psychiatrists cannot get involved in the ordinary course of practice.

Consider the plight of the psychiatrist involved in caring for an opiate-dependent patient who is seeking, or claims to be seeking, admission to a detoxification program but has an admission date that is several days off. What can or should the physician do? It is illegal to prescribe opiates to "sustain an addiction." The best procedure is to consult with the detoxification program staff as to what to do. Under unusual circumstances one could provide the patient with a limited supply of propoxyphene (Darvon), a relatively noneuphoriant opiate, to carry the patient until the admission time, but one must know the patient well and be sure that one is not being tricked or manipulated. Clonidine is an even better alternative. In "medical" addicts—patients who are physically dependent on opiates prescribed for pain relief—it is common to continue the prescription until the patient is admitted to a detoxification unit or chronic pain program.

The newest available maintenance treatment is the opiate antagonist naltrexone (Trexan). This is similar to naloxone (Narcan), the opiate antagonist that has long been available to treat opiate overdose, but naltrexone is much longer acting and available in oral form. Either drug could, in theory, be given orally in large daily doses to create a chronic blockade of opiate receptors, which will reliably block (prevent the euphoriant effects of) heroin or other morphine-like drugs. Naloxone is too weak and short acting orally to be usable. Naltrexone is adequate for the purpose but, to date has had even less popularity with opiate addicts than methadone. However, now that it has recently become available to the clinician, it may find a useful niche in the long-term maintenance treatment of some opiate addicts. For the moment, however, naltrexone is still a drug to be used mainly in special programs and not by general psychiatrists unless they are asked to take over a patient who has already been stabilized on naltrexone in a specialty program. The usual dose is 50 mg a day.

SEDATIVES AND HYPNOTICS

Detoxification

Over the last 40 years, the problem of sedative addiction (physical and psychic dependence) has shifted from almost completely an abuse of short- or intermediate- acting barbiturates (amobarbital, pentobarbital, secobarbital, etc.) to newer hypnotics (glutethimide, methaqualone) or to benzodiazepines (diazepam and others). All of these agents (and alcohol) produce cross-tolerance, that is, physical withdrawal symptoms in a patient dependent on any one of these drugs can be relieved by an adequate dose of another. The time course of withdrawal symptoms differs with the half-lives of the drugs involved, coming on within 12 to 16 hours after the last dose of a barbiturate (e.g., amobarbital) and perhaps two to five days after the last dose of diazepam.

Early withdrawal symptoms include anxiety, restlessness, agitation, nausea, vomiting, and fatigue. Later, weakness develops, often with abdominal cramps plus tachycardia, postural hypotension, hyperreflexia, and gross resting tremor. Insomnia and nightmares may occur. Peak symptoms, including grand mal seizures in some instances, occur at about two to three days after short-acting drugs (amobarbital, lorazepam, alprazolam) and five to 10 days after long-acting drugs (diazepam, clorazepate). Of patients who have seizures, about half will develop delirium with disorientation, anxiety, and visual hallucinations. Even without seizures, patients in benzodiazepine withdrawal may be mildly confused, perceive lights as being too bright and sounds as too loud, get mildly paranoid, and feel depersonalized.

Sedative withdrawal, particularly from barbiturates, can be fatal, and—once it has progressed to delirium—it is not readily reversible. For this reason withdrawal from sedative dependence should be considered a medical emergency, and patients presenting in withdrawal should be treated as such. Withdrawal syndromes from benzodiazepines may be less severe.

In contrast, opiate withdrawal symptoms are rarely life-threatening and always reversible if an opiate is given.

It is probable that regimens could be worked out for using any long-acting sedative such as phenobarbital, chlordiazepoxide, or diazepam to ameliorate withdrawal from sedatives, but we know of no well-developed medication strategy based on this principle. The most commonly recommended regimen uses pentobarbital (Nembutal) to establish the degree of dependence and then converts the patient to phenobarbital for the real detoxification phase.

Pentobarbital Tolerance Test

Once the patient is no longer sedated or intoxicated and is showing early withdrawal symptoms, 200 mg of pentobarbital should be given by mouth and the patient observed one hour later for signs of sedative intoxication. If the patient is asleep at that point, it is likely that no detoxification is necessary because the patient has almost no tolerance to the drug. If the patient has nystagmus, slurred speech, ataxia, or sedation one hour after the initial 200 mg dose, he or she has probably been taking less than the equivalent of 800 mg of pentobarbital a day. This patient can then be stabilized on 100 mg to 200 mg of pentobarbital every six hours, depending on the degree of sedation induced by the initial 200 mg test dose.

If the patient shows no response to the initial 200 mg test dose, he or she requires more than 800 mg a day. To determine the needed dose, the patient should be given 100 mg every two hours until he or she *does* show signs of intoxication (sedation) or until a total dose of 500 mg of pentobarbital in six hours has been given. The total dose given in the first six hours (300 mg to 500 mg) is the patient's six-hour requirement, and this dose *could* be given every six hours and gradually tapered by 100 mg a day.

However, it is better to calculate the initial 24-hour requirement (four times the initial six-hour dose) and convert it to phenobarbital at 30 mg of the latter for each 100 mg of pentobarbital (e.g., 1000 mg a day of pentobarbital requires 300 mg a day of phenobarbital). The daily phenobarbital dose needed should be divided into thirds and given every eight hours for the first 48 hours.

After two days, the phenobarbital dose is decreased by 30

mg a day until the patient is totally withdrawn. Obviously, if the patient appears oversedated on the calculated dose, it could be slightly reduced, or it could be slightly increased in the face of continuing objective signs of withdrawal.

The above program should be used in patients with patterns of *serious* sedative abuse who have been taking doses large enough to lead to frequent sedative intoxication with behavioral consequences (fights, falls, ataxia, job loss, car accidents) or in patients who combine moderate prescribed benzodiazepine doses (e.g., 30 mg a day of diazepam) with excessive alcohol intake.

For the more common psychiatric patient who has become probably physically dependent on prescribed benzodiazepines at *moderate* doses taken for over a year, the benzodiazepine dose can be gradually decreased while the patient is followed as an outpatient, if the patient can tolerate such a program. A shifting from short-acting benzodiazepines, such as lorazepam or alprazolam, to longer acting ones like diazepam or halazepam can be tried if tapering of the shorter acting drug leads to uncomfortable symptoms. It is not clear whether rapid inpatient withdrawal is required in such patients, but it seems legitimate if outpatient withdrawal is poorly tolerated. It may be that slow withdrawal over weeks produces more discomfort than a systematic rapid inpatient regimen.

The other issue here is that mild benzodiazepine withdrawal symptoms should be looked for more carefully in patients admitted to psychiatric hospitals who have had their prior sedative benzodiazepine medication abruptly stopped. A few patients appear to become quite uncomfortable with typical withdrawal symptoms after discontinuation of doses as low as 5 mg of diazepam or 30 mg of flurazepam a day if the doses have been taken regularly for many years. Physicians may forget that sedative withdrawal may be occurring when a depressed or schizophrenic patient begins to get more agitated and may be painfully surprised and discomfited when the patient suddenly has a grand mal seizure.

Alcohol

Ethyl alcohol is a short-acting sedative drug which produces withdrawal syndromes similar to those caused by the barbiturates. The symptoms and signs of withdrawal are as described under sedative detoxification with the caveat that alcoholics either may be very slightly dependent physically but in trouble with alcohol for other reasons or they may be malnourished and/or medically quite ill. Because alcoholism programs tend to treat large numbers of patients, they usually opt for a "standard" detoxification program, which is standard only for a given institution but may differ substantially from one facility to another. King's County Hospital in Brooklyn used paraldehyde routinely and successfully for many years; other sites have used phenobarbital, diazepam, or even antipsychotics such as perphenazine or prochlorperazine.

McLean Hospital has used chlordiazepoxide for at least 15 years; it may be a good choice because it has a long half-life and may be less euphoriant than diazepam. Because of the risk of Wernicke's syndrome in alcoholics, thiamine, 100 mg po or im, must be given on admission. Fifty milligrams a day is given daily thereafter for a month. Chlordiazepoxide is initiated at a maximum of 200 mg per day for the first two days and is reduced by approximately 25 percent per day to zero, with extra doses im or po as needed if the withdrawal symptoms are not adequately controlled.

Phenytoin (Dilantin) is added in patients with a history of withdrawal seizures or in patients unable to give an adequate history. The very rare patient developing delirium tremens despite this regimen should be transferred to a major medical hospital for treatment.

Outpatient detoxification has also been carried out in patients with adequate motivation and an adequate social support system. Here, 25 mg of chlordiazepoxide taken every four hours, or less often if not needed, is probably reasonable for the first day with tapering thereafter (see above). In very tremulous patients who have to be handled as outpatients, a 100 mg im dose of chlordiazepoxide may be indicated. Here the drug's slow absorption from the tissues is an asset, rather than the liability it is in other psychiatric conditions where rapid sedation is the desired effect.

As with opiate withdrawal and maintenance treatment, the general psychiatrist will often be well advised to refer patients to specialized alcoholism programs for, at least, the management of detoxification and possible medical or neurological complications.

Maintenance Treatment

Most alcoholism programs rely mainly on Alcoholics Anonymous plus other educational, psychotherapeutic, and psychosocial modalities. Disulfiram (Antabuse) is often prescribed (or recommended). McLean uses a daily dose of 250 mg for patients over 170 pounds in weight and 125 mg (half a tablet) for patients under that weight. If the disulfiram is taken daily and alcohol is ingested, the following symptoms appear in this general order: flushing, sweating, palpitations, dyspnea, hyperventilation, tachycardia, hypotension, nausea, and vomiting. These events are usually followed by drowsiness and are usually gone after the patient has slept for a period.

Diphenhydramine, 50 mg parenterally, may be helpful in severe disulfiram-alcohol reactions. Hypotension, shock, or arrhythmias are treated symptomatically. Oxygen is useful in respiratory distress. Hypokalemia may occur. Severe reactions require emergency treatment in a medical setting.

Obviously, the willingness to take disulfiram and thereby commit oneself either to stay off alcohol or suffer unpleasant effects if one drinks is a test of motivation to stay dry. It is still, after all these years, not firmly established that the drug is more than a test of motivation or of compliance with therapy. Long-acting injectable disulfiram preparations have been tested abroad, but these are not available in this country.

Disulfiram can cause side effects such as fatigue, a metallic taste, rarely impotence, even more rarely toxic psychosis, and very rarely a severe, occasionally fatal toxic hepatitis. The last named usually comes early in treatment and is the basis for a labeling recommendation that liver function tests be carried out before disulfiram is begun and again after about two weeks.

Metronidazole (Flagyl) has mild disulfiram-like properties and can cause adverse effects when alcohol is taken with it. Studies of the use of metronidazole in alcoholism have been generally negative.

Beyond disulfiram, there is no specific drug therapy for alcoholism, although individual studies have endorsed such diverse drugs as lithium, propranolol, fluoxetine, and chlordiazepoxide, but none of these is well validated as being effective.

Obviously, if a patient has a drug-responsive psychiatric disorder such as major depression in addition to alcoholism, it should be treated appropriately. The treatment of episodic or chronic residual anxiety symptoms after detoxification is a problem. The use of benzodiazepines is usually frowned upon, probably correctly, although a case could be made that chlordiazepoxide could be considered the sedative equivalent of methadone and might be able to be taken at a stable, controlled rate, whereas alcohol, if used to control anxiety, leads to uncontrolled use. Nonabusable alternatives to sedative benzodiazepines in anxious, abstinent alcoholics include propranolol, clonidine, hydroxyzine, tricyclic antidepressants, and buspirone.

Bibliography

Charney D, Sternberg D, Kleber H, et al: The clinical use of clonidine in abrupt withdrawal from methadone. Arch Gen Psychiatry 38:1273–1277, 1981

Cole JO, Ryback RS: Pharmacological therapy, in Alcoholism: Interdisciplinary Approaches to an Enduring Problem. Edited by Tarter R, Sugarman AA. Reading, Mass, Addison-Wesley, 1976, pp 687–734

Ginzburg HM: Naltrexone: Its Clinical Utility [DHHS Publication No (ADM) 84–1358]. Washington, DC, US Government Printing Office, 1984

Mirin S (ed): Substance Abuse and Psychopathology. Washington, DC, American Psychiatric Press, 1984

Shader R (ed): Manual of Psychiatric Therapeutics. Boston, Little, Brown, 1975 [See Chapters 11 through 14]

Smith D, Wesson D: Phenobarbital techniques for treatment of barbiturate dependence. Arch Gen Psychiatry 24:56–60, 1971

Washton A, Resnick R: Clonidine for opiate detoxification: outpatient clinical trial. Am J Psychiatry 137:1121–1122, 1980

Weiss RO, Mirin SM: Intoxication and withdrawal syndromes, in Manual of Psychiatric Emergencies. Edited by Hyman S. Boston, Little, Brown, 1984, pp 217–227

Drugs in Special Situations

Most published reports evaluating the efficacy of psychoactive drugs in psychiatric patients carefully select physically healthy, adult but nonelderly patients. Unfortunately, in clinical practice physicians frequently encounter patients with psychiatric disorders who are also medically ill, pregnant, brain-damaged, elderly, or juveniles but who are otherwise appropriate candidates for conventional pharmacotherapy. This chapter will address some of these problems.

12

PREGNANCY

A markedly manic drug-free patient believed to be in the sixth week of pregnancy was admitted to McLean Hospital a few months ago. She was kept drug-free in seclusion, and often in restraint, for a week because the treating psychiatrist was afraid to initiate neuroleptic treatment for fear of harming the fetus. One of the authors consulted on the case and advised proceeding with haloperidol therapy despite the presumed pregnancy on the grounds that severe hyperactivity and distress were a risk to both patient and fetus, whereas there was no direct evidence that haloperidol or any other neuroleptic leads to any specific birth defect. The physician in charge disagreed. Finally, an ultrasound examination revealed a false pregnancy, and appropriate drug treatment was begun. This case illustrates one kind of clinical dilemma. Thalidomide, with its gross fetal deformities, still haunts all of pharmacotherapy.

As far as we can determine, the only drugs commonly used in psychiatry with proven relationships to specific birth defects are lithium salts and some anticonvulsants, especially phenytoin. Lithium has been associated with cardiac abnormalities, especially Ebstein's anomaly, while anticonvulsants have been associated with a variety of birth defects.

Beyond this, there is no clear evidence that any standard psychiatric drug does (or does not) cause birth defects. Congenital abnormalities occur in babies born to mothers who are taking no drugs at all, but there is a general suspicion that any drug *might* be bad for the fetus, and no doctor feels comfortable recommending drug therapy for a female patient who is believed to have recently become pregnant, or who intends to become pregnant. Of course, whenever possible, drug therapy should be avoided in such instances.

Unfortunately, there are some women with severe, even disabling psychiatric disorders who either wish to become pregnant or actually become pregnant, and a choice must be made between treating the patient and avoiding medicating the fetus. If the situation is not a crisis, as in the patient who is on maintenance medication but would like to become pregnant, outside consultation can be obtained from a dysmorphologist (an expert in birth defects), a type of specialist that can be found in major medical centers. Telephone hot lines providing information on the effects of drugs on the fetus are also available. One of these, the Pregnancy Environmental Hotline (Teratogen Information Service, National

Birth Defect Center), is located at the Kennedy Memorial Hospital in Brighton, Massachusetts. Its telephone number is (617) 787–4957. Staff members are willing to accept calls and refer callers to other programs around the country when appropriate. Two major reference works in this area are listed in the bibliography of this chapter.

The information from the dysmorphologist or the telephone hot line will tell you whether there is any solid evidence that a particular drug is teratogenic, but it will not solve the clinician's whole problem. The final decision has to be based on the seriousness of the patient's distress and the reasonableness of the desire to have a child. Informed consent from the patient and her family (including her husband or her parents, when appropriate) for the treatment plan are necessary whether one decides to leave the patient drug-free with the risks of that course, or whether one decides to continue with a needed medication despite the pregnancy.

If one can avoid medication for the first three months of pregnancy, then the risk of fetal abnormality is much reduced, but other risks can occur. Babies born to mothers who are physically dependent on sedatives or opiates will suffer withdrawal syndromes and will need to be treated postnatally. We have heard a rumor of a baby being born with a dystonic reaction when the mother had been on neuroleptics, and autonomic withdrawal symptoms presumably could occur in the newborn if the mother has been on tricyclic antidepressants. One can justify withdrawing medication carefully from pregnant women a few weeks before delivery.

After the baby is born, nursing mothers on medication will probably excrete drug in breast milk. In the absence of data on breast milk concentrations of a specific drug, it is hard to estimate the seriousness of this problem, but generally breast milk concentrations are lower than drug levels in the blood and the total dose ingested by the infant may be quite small. If a reliable laboratory procedure is available for the drug the mother is receiving, the actual drug levels in the mother's milk can be determined. There is a general belief that mothers on lithium should not nurse their babies.

A higher and more diffuse level of concern is the possibility that drug therapy with a psychoactive drug during pregnancy (or nursing) may somehow affect brain development in the child. There are really no data on which to base concern or with which to reassure the patient.

As with many unponderable risk-benefit situations in medicine, the suffering or psychiatric hospitalization of the mother must be weighed against the often unknown risk to the infant as interpreted by the doctor, patient, and patient's family.

CHILDREN AND ADOLESCENTS

Prepubescent children have efficient livers. This generally allows them to metabolize drugs rapidly and enables them to tolerate somewhat higher doses of psychiatric drugs per unit of weight than adults tolerate. After puberty drug metabolism resembles that seen in young adults. The lesson here, of course, is not that seven-year-olds should be given huge doses of drugs but that they should be started on very small doses. If there is no response, the dose may be gradually increased to adult dosages, adjusted for weight, without fear of unusual toxicity of conventional kinds.

On the other hand, there are no studies at all of the long-term consequences of psychiatric drug therapy in childhood on brain function, behavior, or physical health in adult life. The decision to use a drug treatment for a psychiatrically ill child or young adolescent must therefore be based on a clear and urgent clinical need. The psychiatric disorder must pose significant danger to the child's development and well-being and should only be undertaken after considered medical and psychiatric evaluation.

It should be noted that most standard psychiatric drugs

have not received FDA approval for "use" in children or even in adolescents, mainly because the necessary studies have not been carried out.

Stimulants

The best studied and best validated drug therapy for psychiatrically ill children is the use of stimulants—*d*-amphetamine, methylphenidate, and magnesium pemoline (see Chapter 8)—in attentional deficit disorder. Caffeine is not effective in this condition; tricyclic antidepressants (e.g., desipramine) in low dosages (10-75 mg a day) may also be useful but act more slowly. Stimulants often show effects in hours; tricyclic antidepressants may take days or weeks. Research on the effects of stimulants on various kinds of behavior suggests that the drug effects are complex. The dose that controls overactivity best may be too high for optimal improvement in learning. The stimulants may cause slight decrease in body growth, perhaps 1-3 cm in height over the entire developmental period. Children on stimulants may show side effects such as anorexia, insomnia, dysphoria, even tics. On the other hand, some children with attention deficit disorder are markedly benefitted, generally more in behavior than in academic performance, whereas others are somewhat better and a few are not benefitted or even become more agitated. Of the available stimulants, *d*-amphetamine and methylphenidate are a bit more effective and safer than magnesium pemoline. Magnesium pemoline can cause hepatocellular damage, presumably due to toxic metabolites, in 1-3 percent of children treated. Monthly tests of liver function are in order if magnesium pemoline is used.

Some children respond better, unpredictably, to one of the three stimulants than to the other two. *d*-Amphetamine has the advantage of being generally cheaper. It is worth trying patients with a good stimulant response off medication every few months to see if the drug is still needed. The practice of only giving a child with attention deficit disorder medication on school days may have the disadvantage of impairing the child's family and peer relationships as well as learning outside the school situation. Some children continue to benefit from stimulants into adolescence or even adulthood. Dosage may need to be adjusted over time as the child grows and matures.

Antipsychotics

In autistic or psychotic children, neuroleptics are often used with some benefit. These conditions in children under 15 rarely show marked improvement on antipsychotics, although some decrease in overactive, disorganized behavior can occur. There is no evidence that children are any less tolerant of these drugs than are adults, except perhaps for an even higher rate of dystonia early in treatment in adolescents. However, the risk of tardive dyskinesia and the lower likelihood of marked improvement make it necessary that clinicians use these agents cautiously, document carefully the clinical effects observed, and periodically assess the patient off medication to make sure the treatment is really useful as a maintenance therapy. In older adolescents, acute psychotic syndromes begin to resemble those seen in adults and may be treated in the same manner (see Chapter 4).

Antipsychotics in low dosages (e.g., 0.5-3 mg of haloperidol a day) can also control the tics of Tourette's disorder; clonidine has also been reported to be helpful in severe cases of this disorder. Antipsychotics have often been used to control the behavior of angry, impulsive children and adolescents without psychosis. The risks and benefits of this use are unclear. Sedative antihistamines (diphenhydramine, hydroxyzine) should be tried first. If antipsychotics are used, 10-50 mg of chlorpromazine one to four times a day may be more useful than the same total dose at bedtime and more useful than the high potency, less sedative neuroleptics. But continued use of these potentially harmful drugs to control deviant behavior is hard to justify unless it can be clearly shown that, for each particular patient, the drug makes a major and clinically important difference.

The side effects of antipsychotics, including tardive dyskinesia, are essentially the same in children as in adults. However, the possibility of cognitive blunting with these drugs may be relatively more of a problem in children. An inert child who is not learning or functioning may be less trouble to others but may develop more normally if medication is reduced or stopped.

Antidepressants

Tricyclic antidepressants are effective in the treatment of enuresis at doses of 0.3-1.0 mg/kg of imipramine or equivalent drugs, but behavioral treatments are generally preferred because they are also effective and may have a lower relapse rate. Attention deficit disorder tends to respond in the same dosage range. Monoamine oxidase inhibitors are said also to be effective in both these conditions, but their use is not well studied.

Some children clearly meet conventional adult criteria for major depressive disorder and respond to tricyclic antidepressants. Food and Drug Administration guidelines recommend an upper dosage limit of 2.5 mg/kg; however, some studies report dosages up to 5.0 mg/kg as often being necessary for clinical response. Monitoring of cardiac function is wise when tricyclics are used in children, with EKGs being done prior to starting therapy, again when the dose exceeds 3 mg/kg, and then every two weeks if dosage is being increased. Significant slowing of cardiac conduction (P-R interval over 0.20, QRS interval over 0.12) may require lowering the dose. Side effects in children resemble those seen in adults. Blood level monitoring is about as useful as it is in adults. Imipramine is the best studied drug, and positive correlations between blood level and improvement are often found in clinical trials.

Local experience suggests that depressive symptoms in adolescents rarely include major appetite changes or early morning awakening. Overly sound and lengthy sleep with dysphoria on awakening are more common. Physical symptoms, fatigue, irritability, anger, and retardation for the first few hours in the day may be present without subjective recognition of depression or sadness. Sex drive is decreased. These adolescents often have a family history of affective disorder. This pattern often responds to tricyclic therapy, although formal controlled studies have not been done. Panic agoraphobia can occur in adolescents and can be treated with antidepressants.

Lithium

Adolescents can show a typical bipolar picture that can respond to lithium therapy. Preadolescent children rarely show mania but can show cyclic mood and behavior shifts with periods of impulsivity, social intrusiveness, tantrums, mood lability, and nonpsychotic euphoria with parallel shifts in vegetative symptoms, which sometimes respond to lithium. The side effects of lithium are the same in children as in adults. To date, no one knows the long-term consequences of long-term maintenance lithium treatment begun in childhood or adolescence.

Antianxiety Drugs

Benzodiazepines are sometimes of use for short periods in pavor nocturnis or sleep walking. If used for daytime anxiety, they can increase activity and produce or aggravate behavior disorders. Severe school phobia is better treated with imipramine, although a single dose of a benzodiazepine may be used occasionally to allay anticipatory anxiety and help a child return to a feared situation for the first time.

Sedative antihistamines are believed to have some antianxiety or hypnotic utility in children for short periods. Prolonged use could lead to anticholinergic side effects and cognitive impairment.

It is worth remembering that newer drugs are rarely studied in children or adolescents prior to marketing, and even the older drugs are often only partially studied. The place of drug therapy in children and adolescents is still controversial. Drugs should be reserved for clearly distressed or dysfunctional conditions where psychosocial treatments either have failed or are only likely to be of short-term benefit. Drug therapy needs to be carefully monitored and requires close collaboration between the physician, the parents, and often school personnel or other caretakers. Prolonged maintenance drug therapy is sometimes justifiable, but there should be strong clinical evidence of benefit, and trials off medication are often indicated to make sure the drug is still making a useful difference.

GERIATRIC PATIENTS

Elderly psychiatric patients present a variety of potential problems for the psychiatrist considering prescribing psychoactive drugs. The elderly may have decreased ability to metabolize some drugs, although this has been documented only infrequently. They *may* have low serum protein levels, which could lead them to have relatively higher levels of free drug (not bound to protein) at any given blood level; free drug is usually presumed to be more active and more likely to cross the blood-brain barrier. The elderly *may* be more sensitive to peripheral side effects (e.g., hypotension, constipation) than younger patients at the same dose or blood level. They *may* also be more prone to central side effects (e.g., delirium, tremor, tardive dyskinesia). None of these presumptions are well documented except for delirium and tardive dyskinesia, chiefly because no adequate studies have been done.

Probably the elderly have a reduced reserve of both brain function and cardiovascular competence, which leaves them more vulnerable to drug side effects. In addition, the consequences of side effects, such as falls due to orthostatic hypotension, falls due to confusion, or ataxia or decubitus ulcers due to prolonged oversedation, are more likely to be serious in the elderly. The situation is made worse by the higher likelihood of coexisting medical illness and the use of other drugs for these illnesses in the elderly as well as by the lack of any clear criteria for predicting which elderly patients need very low, cautious dosage regimens of psychoactive drugs and which patients will require (and tolerate) rather large dosages to attain adequate treatment response.

For the standard psychiatric conditions such as depression, mania, chronic schizophrenia, generalized anxiety disorder, etc., the only safe and reasonable approach is to begin with very low drug dosages and to increase the dosage cautiously. As an example, 25 mg of imipramine or trimipramine at bedtime is a reasonable starting dose for healthy patients over 60, and a 10 mg dose is reasonable for patients over 70 or for patients over 60 with concurrent medical problems or with evidence of organic dementia. In such patients, dosage increments should occur every three to seven days, not every day, so that the clinician has a chance to assess side effects before increasing the dose. Other antidepressants, such as trazodone and monoamine oxidase inhibitors, and ECT have been used effectively in elderly patients with major depressions. The difference is not in choice of drug but in the caution with which dosage is increased and side effects are monitored.

Another presumption in the treatment of elderly patients is that anticholinergic drugs increase the likelihood of delirium. On this basis, desipramine should be safer than amitriptyline and fluphenazine safer than thioridazine. Our review of the literature on tricyclic use in the elderly suggests, however, that delirium more often occurs in patients on a tricyclic-neuroleptic combination and that this side effect can be transient and relatively easily managed. Again, there are no adequate controlled trials documenting this issue.

If benzodiazepines are to be used as hypnotics or for daytime anxiety, again use the lowest dose (e.g., 2 mg of diazepam or 0.125 mg of triazolam) first to see whether this dose is adequate and to make sure side effects do not occur. There is evidence that benzodiazepine metabolism is slowed in the elderly and a presumption that higher, cumulative blood levels will be associated with behavioral toxicity. Occasionally, elderly (and young adult) patients will complain of excessive morning sedation after slowly metabolized hypnotics like flurazepam, but there is a good deal of individual variability in the extent to which this consequence of slowed metabolism actually causes demonstrable clinical problems.

Lithium excretion is, on the average, slowed in the elderly as a consequence of an age-related decrease in kidney function. Therefore, older patients should be started on low doses— 300 mg a day in patients in their 60s and early 70s and 150 mg a day (half a tablet) in patients who are older. Lithium levels and clinical signs of toxicity should be watched for scrupulously. It is our impression that the elderly can slip from therapeutic to toxic blood levels more rapidly and insidiously than young adult patients. On the other hand, lithium can be as effective in some older bipolar patients as in younger ones, although some elderly patients with a late onset may have a simultaneous organic disorder that does not respond well to lithium.

In older chronic schizophrenics, there is a belief that lower antipsychotic dosages are needed than in younger adult patients. There is, again, no real evidence that this is true, but cautious attempts at gradually tapering dosage are indicated in schizophrenic patients over 60 who are on maintenance neuroleptic treatment. When such patients have stopped their medication and become acutely psychotic, cautious low-dosage medication (e.g., 1-2 mg a day of haloperidol or fluphenazine) should be tried for the first week to see if a clinical response can be obtained without resorting to high dosages. However, if the patient fails to improve and has a history of requiring and tolerating higher neuroleptic dosage, the dose can be gradually raised, again watching for side effects. The use of antiparkinsonian drugs *could* cause delirium, but leaving the patient with dystonia or pseudoparkinsonism is equally undesirable; the clinician is forced to feel his way, attempting to maximize benefit and minimize adverse effects. This applies equally to the use of neuroleptics in younger adult patients, but—in the elderly—the problems encountered in attempting to achieve the right balance of medications may be more frequent.

Tardive dyskinesia is statistically more prevalent in elderly patients, especially women, on maintenance neuroleptics, but in chronic schizophrenic patients the dyskinesia has usually already been present for years and is not a contraindication to using neuroleptics to achieve relief of psychotic symptoms. In the rare chronic patient showing new dyskinesia, a trial off neuroleptics is usually indicated. The concurrent presence of both pseudoparkinsonism and dyskinesia in the same patient is more common in the elderly.

DEMENTED ELDERLY PATIENTS

Most elderly patients with mild, moderate, or severe dementia have Alzheimer's disease, although some have multi-infarct dementia, a few have both, and some have neither. The best treatment for dementia is to diagnose a treatable, reversible cause such as vitamin deficiency, hypothyroidism, or congestive heart failure and to treat the underlying medical condition. The other confounding diagnosis is pseudodementia secondary to major depression. Some authors believe that depression can, in fact, cause dementia in the elderly, and depression can certainly aggravate mild, preexisting cognitive dysfunction. The evidence is clear that depression should be carefully and thoroughly treated when cognitive impairment and depression coexist and that antidepressants should also be used in patients with strokes or organic mood lability even if the depressive syndrome is only partially present. The odds favor a substantial improvement over any worsening of organic deficit, although dosage should be started low and raised cautiously. It *is* clear that patients with behavioral deficits due to strokes who show insomnia, weight loss, agitation, and inability to participate in rehabilitative programs can do well on tricyclic antidepressants and presumably on other antidepressants. Just because the dysphoria *seems* appropriate to the disability, treatment should not be withheld.

Dementia alone is no indication, to date, for drug therapy. The only drug marketed in the United States for senile symptoms, ergoloid mesylates (Hydergine), does seem to regularly be a bit more effective than placebo in a large number of double-blind, placebo-controlled studies, but the effects are weak, different in different studies and usually only manifest after two to three months, making the marginal utility of this treatment questionable. A variety of drugs have been studied in dementia, including piracetam, vincamine, lecithin, oral physostigmine, etc., but so far none has been shown to be regularly and safely useful.

Patients with chronic dementia sometimes show agitation, irascibility, night-wandering, paranoid ideation, or hallucinations and become major management problems at home or in psychiatric hospitals or nursing homes. Many of these patients are routinely treated with neuroleptics, often with dubious benefit. The most recent review of the few controlled studies in this area suggests that only a third of these patients are clearly benefitted by low-dose neuroleptics. In our own experience thioridazine is not better tolerated than low doses of more potent antipsychotics; all neuroleptics show an unfortunate tendency to cause pseudoparkinsonism and akathisia in the elderly. These, plus the increased risk of tardive dyskinesia and the probably increased risk of organic confusional states when antiparkinsonian drugs are added, make neuroleptics often unsatisfactory drugs in agitated, demented patients. Sometimes they are very helpful, but more often the side effects limit their usefulness. They tend to be overused because clinicians believe they lack other options.

Other options are, in fact, limited, but psychosocial measures should be tried and neuroleptic therapy should be tapered and stopped from time to time to make sure that it is actually helping. Alternative drug therapies such as propranolol, lithium, carbamazepine, diphenhydramine, and lorazepam (see Chapters 4 and 5) might be helpful in occasional patients, although all can cause side effects and must be used with caution. Better studies of more kinds of drug therapy are needed in this area, but in their absence clinicians have to cautiously try to do their best with such measures as are available.

MENTAL RETARDATION

As with the demented elderly, the institutionalized mentally retarded have been treated routinely for decades with neuroleptics, mainly thioridazine, for a wide range of behavioral disorders. Court decisions have mandated evaluation of such patients off medications, and it now appears that only a fraction of those receiving long-term neuroleptic medication are clinically better on them than off them. The neuroleptic-responsive retarded patients have not been well characterized, but it seems probable that some show psychotic symptoms that would qualify for a diagnosis of schizophrenia.

Recent papers document the existence of depressive and bipolar disorders manifesting somewhat atypically in relatively or completely nonverbal patients. Such patients are appropriate candidates for treatment with standard antidepressants or lithium. Under special circumstances the less well studied drugs such as carbamazepine, valproic acid, or propranolol may be worth cautious use (see Chapters 4 and 5). In retarded or nonretarded patients with a seizure disorder, there is a worry that psychiatric drugs, including tricyclic antidepressants and neuroleptics, may lower the seizure threshold and increase the likelihood or rate of convulsions. There is no firm evidence in this area. Maprotiline, imipramine, and amitriptyline have been more often connected with seizure occurrence in nonretarded depressed patients in our experience, but these are, or were, also the most commonly used tricyclics in the McLean Hospital system at the time seizures were seen. Trazodone is least likely to affect seizure threshold. Bupropion has been associated with seizures. Within the neuroleptics there is a belief that haloperidol or molindone is least likely to affect seizure occurrence. In our experience chlorpromazine and loxapine are occasionally associated with seizure occurrence.

In patients with a known seizure disorder that is adequately treated with anticonvulsants, it is relatively unlikely that any of the standard psychiatric drugs will make a clinically important difference in seizure frequency. In retarded patients on phenytoin, phenobarbital or primidone for seizure control, there is a real possibility that the seizure medication may be causing cognitive dysfunction. It may be worth shifting the patient to carbamazepine to see if the patient may function better on that relatively different medication.

Stimulants may also be worth a trial in hyperactive retarded patients who are under close clinical observation. Stimulants have the advantage of causing clear clinical effects (improvement or worsening) within a few hours or days of reaching an adequate dose so that the trials of a stimulant may be completed in one or two weeks.

MEDICAL CONDITIONS

Some psychiatric syndromes are caused by or strongly associated with medical disorders. Others are commonly associated with medications used to treat medical or neurological conditions. On the other hand, some medical conditions and some drugs used to treat medical conditions complicate the use of standard psychoactive drugs to treat coexisting psychiatric disorders.

Psychiatric Disorders from Medical Illness

Psychiatric disorders, especially depression, can occur with and are presumably caused by thyroid or adrenal cortical dysfunction, uremia, cancer of the pancreas, and any metastatic carcinomatosis sufficiently often to make it worth ascertaining that these conditions do not exist in depressed patients. Other more obvious conditions such as strokes, multiple sclerosis, lupus erythematosus and Parkinson's disease are often associated with depression, as well as with organic brain disorders. Chronic pain syndromes including headache and low-back pain are so confounded with depressive syndromes that primary antidepressant therapy is often indicated. For some medical conditions such as hypothyroidism, treating the underlying condition is the first order of business. For others, the presence of an untreatable medical or neurological condition does not contraindicate, per se, standard antidepressant therapy.

Hyperthyroidism, caffeinism, hypoglycemia, paroxysmal tachycardias, and pheochromocytoma can all mimic panic disorder and should be ruled out. A medical reevaluation is indicated if standard drug therapies fail or atypical features exist.

Psychiatric Disorders Associated with Medical Drugs

A variety of antihypertensive drugs (e.g., propranolol, reserpine, alpha-methyl-dopa) can sometimes precipitate depression. Shifting to a thiazide diuretic or a different, non-centrally acting beta-blocker (e.g., atenolol) can be helpful, or a tricyclic antidepressant alone can sometimes adequately treat both the depression and the hypertension.

Diazepam has also occasionally been associated with increased depression. Both benzodiazepines and barbiturates can aggravate attentional deficit disorder, and stimulants can aggravate schizophrenia or mania.

Steroids and L-dopa can mimic almost any known psychiatric syndrome including delirium, paranoid psychosis, mania, depression, and anxiety.

The whole range of drugs used in Parkinson's disease can cause hallucinosis and confusion. Sometimes anticholinergic drugs used in gastrointestinal disorders can also cause anticholinergic confusion and delirium, as can digitalis-like drugs and cimetidine-like agents.

It is impossible to list or predict all the drugs or drug combinations which at some dose in some patient can elicit or aggravate symptoms of psychiatric disorder. In patients receiving several drugs for medical conditions who present with depression, anxiety, or psychosis coming on after the drugs were begun, a careful reevaluation of the patient's pharmacotherapies is necessary. Stopping the less obviously crucial medications and shifting to less centrally active alternative drugs where some medication is necessary are reasonable steps.

Psychiatric Disorders Complicated by Medical Disorders

Some medical disorders should have reasonably predictable effects on the pharmacokinetics of standard psychiatric drugs if enough were known to understand what should be happening. In the case of kidney failure and lithium therapy, the facts are clear. If renal clearance is decreased, lithium excretion will be decreased in a reasonably proportionate manner. In patients with substantially elevated serum creatinine and blood urea nitrogen who are not in acute renal failure, very small doses of lithium (e.g., 150 mg a day) can be cautiously begun and titrated in the same way that one would in a healthy patient but more cautiously and with smaller increments. Here lithium citrate given in milliliter doses could give extra flexibility. We have heard of a patient on renal dialysis who was stabilized on lithium by having a single 300 mg dose given after each episode of dialysis. This maintained an adequate blood level until the next dialysis removed the lithium ions.

With liver damage, the effects are more complicated. Most drugs are partially destroyed in the liver after absorption from the small intestine (the first-pass effect). When liver tissue is damaged, many drugs will get into the general circulation at much higher relative levels. Usually glucuronidation as a method of drug deactivation is well preserved while demethylation and other metabolic processes are more readily impaired. This is why drugs like diazepam, which need to be demethylated, cause much higher blood levels per unit dose in cirrhosis, whereas drugs like lorazepam, which are only glucuronidated, are handled normally. Unfortunately, it is not always clear to even a skilled clinical pharmacologist exactly what the effect of chronic liver disease on the clinical actions of any particular drug will be. It is likely that standard tricyclics such as amitriptyline and imipramine will be less readily converted to their desmethyl metabolites, nortriptyline or desipramine, in patients with partial liver failure. The consequences of this shift—perhaps more sedation, confusion, or anticholinergic side effects— are less clear. The obvious lesson is to proceed very cautiously, to use blood level determinations, if available, and to assume that liver damage will markedly increase a drug's half-life, making gradual accumulation of higher and higher blood levels quite possible over a couple of weeks at a constant daily dose. Lowered blood protein levels, common in liver disease, may also increase free drug levels, unbound to protein, making a drug more potent at lower total blood levels measured in the conventional manner.

An "overactive" liver can also pose problems. Some known drugs, including barbiturates, phenytoin, and cigarette smoking, will induce hepatic enzymes and will increase the rate at which some psychiatric drugs are destroyed, making higher dosages necessary to achieve clinical results (see Chapters 3, 5, and 9). It is also worth noting that even drug-free patients can show large degrees of biological variability in their natural rates of drug metabolism. As an example, Glassman et al. (1977; in Chapter 3) found imipramine levels to vary from 40 to 1040 ng/ml in depressed patients receiving 2.5 mg/kg of imipramine. Again, the lesson is that patients on other drugs for medical reasons may well have altered response based either on increased or decreased hepatic metabolism of the psychiatric drug that has just been added (not to mention pharmacologic interactions such as additive sedation or additive postural hypotension). In the likely absence of clear knowledge as to the interactions in a particular patient of, say, cimetidine, phenytoin, chlorthiazide, and isoniazid with imipramine, the clinician adding imipramine in a patient on all these other drugs must be prepared to proceed cautiously but to use high dosages of imipramine if neither side effects nor clinical response occurs, if blood levels are low, and if electrocardiographic changes are not seen.

In cardiac patients there has long been a fear that all tricyclic antidepressants are cardiotoxic and likely to cause disastrous arrhythmias. This has now been shown quite clearly to be true *only* if the drugs are taken in overdose. The mechanism by which the tricyclics and maprotiline affect cardiac function is by a quinidine-like slowing of cardiac conduction. Tricyclics have, in fact, an ability to decrease cardiac irritability and suppress premature contractions. They are therefore *not* contraindicated in ordinary dosages in depressed patients with premature ventricular contractions and may well help both the cardiac irritability and the depression. The tricyclics should, however, be used with caution in patients with preexisting conduction defects, such as bundle-branch block, and should not be given to patients already on cardiac antiarrhythmic drugs, which act by slowing cardiac conduction since additive effects on conduction could be harmful. Not all cardiologists are aware of the cardiac effects of tricyclics, and the psychiatrist who collaborates with cardiologists or primary care physicians may need to do some educating of his or her consultants.

The other antidepressant with a possible effect on cardiac irritability is trazodone. It does not affect conduction but has occasionally, not regularly, been associated with an increase in premature ventricular contractions and should be avoided in patients with runs of PVCs or ventricular bigemini. Monoamine oxidase inhibitors, in therapeutic dosages, do not have obvious direct effects on cardiac conduction.

The more significant effect of tricyclics and MAOIs is postural hypotension, which can be aggravated (potentiated) in patients already on drugs such as propranolol, which are likely to cause hypotension as well. Although patients with known stable cardiac disease, but not in congestive failure, probably tolerate antidepressants well, patients on multiple cardiac drugs are probably prone to this and other cardiac side effects. For seriously ill cardiac patients with severe depression, electroconvulsive therapy may be the treatment of choice.

Another predictable interaction between psychiataric and general medical drugs is the additive effects of anticholinergic agents such as propantheline (Pro-Banthine), glycopyrrolate (Robinul), or preparations like Donnatal, which contain atropine and scopolamine as well as phenobarbital, or tincture of belladonna. It is possible that the adding of a potent anticholinergic such as amitriptyline to anticholinergic anti-spasmodics could result in urinary retention or paralytic ileus. Additive central anticholinergic effects could cause confusion or delirium. Here glycopyrrolate, which does not cross the blood-brain barrier, would be preferred to atropine if both an anticholinergic tricyclic and an anticholinergic antispasmodic were really needed at the same time.

Other additive or antagonistic interactions probably occur. Some of the better documented ones are discussed in earlier chapters focusing on specific drug classes.

It would be helpful if our current knowledge of drug actions could be put to precise clinical use in assessing the effects of adding a new psychiatric drug to a preexisting melange of medical and psychiatric drugs. Unfortunately drugs do not work like sums in an algebraic equation. One would think, for example, that *d*-amphetamine, an indirect dopamine agonist, would have its action opposed by haloperidol, a reasonably pure dopamine blocking drug. In practice some patients will feel more lively and functional when *d*-amphetamine is added to haloperidol without becoming more psychotic. In practice drugs usually act on several receptors and on both pre- and postsynaptic receptors of a single type, leading to potentially complex effects and interactions. The clinician is often faced with treating, say, schizophrenia, agoraphobia with panic, or depression in a patient with several medical problems requiring concomitant drug therapies likely to influence the metabolism or absorption of a psychiatric drug or to have additive or antagonistic or, more likely, unknown effects in combination with the most appropriate psychiatric drug treatment. All drug therapy consists of a series of empirical clinical trials; medically ill patients simply present more complicated empirical trials. The psychiatrist can try to guess at the more probable ways in which the new drug will act or be affected by the patient's medical disease and ongoing drug therapies, but it is likely to be only guesswork. If there are semipredictable adverse interactions, one can try to either avoid them by choosing the psychiatric drug least likely to cause trouble or can proceed cautiously with close monitoring of the patient for predictable and unpredictable side effects in collaboration with the physicians managing the patient's nonpsychiatric disorders. One worries that medically ill patients will be very fragile and easily become toxic on psychiatric drugs, but it is likely that this is not a general problem—some patients may develop problems while others will tolerate psychiatric drugs unusally well. The reported use of huge haloperidol doses (e.g., 10 mg iv every hour for many hours) in medical or surgical intensive care units makes one wonder whether some seriously ill patients may not be very tolerant of some psychiatric drugs.

Bibliography

Ananth J: Side effects in the neonate from psychotropic agents excreted through breast feeding. Am J Psychiatry 135:801–805, 1978

Barkley R, Cunningham L: Do stimulant drugs improve academic performance of hyperkinetic children? A review of outcome studies. Clin Pediatr (Phila) 17:85–92, 1978

Breunning SE, Ferguson DG, Davidson NA, et al: Effects of thioridazine on the intellectual performance of mentally retarded drug responders and non-responders. Arch Gen Psychiatry 40:309–313, 1983

Briggs G, Bodendorfer T, Freeman R, et al: Drugs in pregnancy and lactation: a reference guide to fetal and neonatal risk. Baltimore, Williams and Wilkins, 1983

Campell M: Psychopharmacology in childhood psychosis. International Journal of Mental Health 4:238–254, 1975

Campbell M: Psychopharmacology, in Basic Handbook of Child Psychiatry. Edited by Noshpitz J, Harrison S. New York, Basic Books, 1979, pp 376–409

Cohen DJ, Detlor J, Young JG, et al: Clonidine ameliorates Gilles de la Tourette's syndrome. Arch Gen Psychiatry 37:1350–1357, 1980

Cole J, Hardy P, Marcel B, et al: Organic states, in Common Treatment Problems in Depression. Edited by Schatzberg A. Washington, DC, American Psychiatric Press, 1985, pp 79–100

Creasey W: Drug disposition in humans. New York, Oxford University Press, 1979

DeLong GR, Nieman GW: Lithium-induced behavior changes in children with symptoms suggesting manic-depressive illness. Psychopharmacol Bull 19:258–265, 1983

DiGiacomo J: The hypertensive or cardiac patient, in Common Treatment Problems in Depression. Edited by Schatzberg A. Washington, DC, American Psychiatric Press, 1985, pp 29–56

Eisendorfer C, Fann WE (eds): Psychopharmacology and Aging. New York, Plenum, 1973

Friedel R: Pharmacokinetics in the geropsychiatric patient, in Psychopharmacology: A Generation of Progress. Edited by Lipton M, DiMascio A, Killam K. New York, Raven Press, 1978, pp 1499–1506

Gastfriend DR, Biederman J, Jellinek MS: Desipramine in the treatment of adolescents with attention deficit disorders. Am J Psychiatry 141:906–908, 1984

Gittelman-Klein R, Klein DF: Controlled imipramine treatment of school phobia. Arch Gen Psychiatry 25:204–207, 1971

Glassman A: The newer antidepressant drugs and their cardiovascular effects. Psychopharmacol Bull 20:272–277, 1984

Glassman A, Walsh B, Roose S, et al: Factors related to orthostatic hypotension associated with tricyclic antidepressants. J Clin Psychiatry 43:35–40, 1982

Gold M, Estroff T, Pottash A: Substance-induced organic mental disorders, in Psychiatry Update, vol 4. Edited by Hales R, Frances A. Washington, DC, American Psychiatric Press, 1985, pp 227–240

Goldberg H, DiMascio A: Psychotropic drugs in pregnancy, in Psychopharmacology: A Generation of Progress. Edited by Lipton M, DiMascio A, Killam K. New York, Raven Press, 1978, pp 1047–1055

Greenblatt D, Shader R: Psychotropic drugs in the general hospital, in Manual of Psychiatric Therapeutics. Edited by Shader R. Boston, Little, Brown, 1975, pp 1–26

Gualtieri CT, Barnhill J, McGimsey J, et al: Tardive dyskinesia and other movement disorders in children treated with psychotropic drugs. J Am Acad Child Psychiatry 19:491–510, 1980

Helms PM: Efficacy of antipsychotics in the treatment of the behavioral complications of dementia: a review of the literature. J Am Geriatr Soc 33:206–209, 1985

Huessey H, Ruoff P: Towards a rational drug usage in a state institution for retarded individuals. Psychiatr J Univ Ottawa 9:56–58, 1984

Lipsey J, Robinson R, Pearlsen J, et al: Nortriptyline treatment of post-stroke depression. Lancet 1:297–300, 1984

Mikkelsen E, Rapoport J: Enuresis: psychopathology, sleep stage and drug response. Urol Clin North Am 1:361–375, 1980

Morgan MH, Read AE: Antidepressants and liver disease. Gut 13:697–701, 1972

Paykel E, Fleminger R, Watson J: Psychiatric side effects of antihypertensive drugs. J Clin Psychopharmacology 2:14–33, 1982

Petti T, Law W: Imipramine treatment of depressed children: a double-blind pilot study. J Clin Psychopharmacol 2:107–110, 1982

Popper CW: Child and adolescent psychopharmacology, in Psychiatry. Edited by Cavenor JO. Philadelphia, Lipppincott, 1985

Prien RF: Chemotherapy in chronic organic brain syndrome: a review of the literature. Psychopharmacol Bull 9:5–20, 1973

Raskin DE: Antipsychotic medications and the elderly. J Clin Psychiatry 46(no 5, sec 2):36–40, 1985

Reisberg B, Ferris SH, Gershon S: An overview of pharmacologic treatment of cognitive decline in the elderly. Am J Psychiatry 138:593–600, 1981

Salzman CA: A primer of geriatric psychopharmacology. Am J Psychiatry 139:67–74, 1982

Shader RI (ed): Psychiatric Complications of Medical Drugs. New York, Raven Press, 1972

Shapiro AK, Shapiro E, Wayne H: Treatment of Tourette's syndrome. Arch Gen Psychiatry 28:92–97, 1973

Shepard TH: The Catalogue of Teratogenic Agents, 4th ed. Baltimore, Johns Hopkins University Press, 1983

Sovner R, Hurley A: Do the mentally retarded suffer from affective illness? Arch Gen Psychiatry 40:61–67, 1983

Thompson TL, Moran MG, Nies AS: Psychotropic drug use in the elderly [Part 2]. N Engl J Med 308:194–199, 1985

Tsuang MM, Lu L, Stotsky BA, et al: Haloperidol vs thioridazine for hospitalized psychogeriatric patients: double-blind study. J Am Geriatr Soc 19:593–600, 1971

Werry JS (ed): Pediatric Psychopharmacology. New York, Brunner/ Mazel, 1978

SUGGESTED READING LIST

Clinicians' Source Materials

Baldessarini RJ: Biomedical Aspects of Depression and Its Treatment. Washington, DC, American Psychiatric Press, 1983

Baldessarini RJ: Chemotherapy in Psychiatry: Principles and Practice. Cambridge, Harvard University Press, 1985

Cole JO (ed): Psychopharmacology Update. Lexington, Collamore Press, 1980

Gilman AG, Goodman LS, Gilman A (eds): Goodman and Gilman's The Pharmacological Basis of Therapeutics, 6th ed. New York, Macmillan, 1980

Hyman SE (ed): Manual of Psychiatric Emergencies. Boston, Little, Brown, 1984

Jefferson JW, Greist JH, Ackerman DL, et al: Lithium Encyclopedia for Clinical Practice, 2nd ed. Washington, DC, American Psychiatric Press, 1986

Klein DF, Davis JM: Diagnosis and Drug Treatment of Psychiatric Disorders. Baltimore, Williams and Wilkins, 1969

Klein DF, Gittleman-Klein R, Quitkin F, et al: Diagnosis and Treatment of Psychiatric Disorders: Adults and Children. Baltimore, Williams and Wilkins, 1980

Lipton M, DiMascio A, Killam KF: Psychopharmacology: A Generation of Progress. New York, Raven Press, 1978

Mason AS, Granacher RPL: Clinical Handbook of Antipsychotic Drug Therapy. New York, Brunnel/Mazel, 1980

For Patients and Families

The American Psychiatric Association's Psychiatric Glossary, 5th ed. Washington, DC, American Psychiatric Association, 1980

Andreasen NC: The Broken Brain: The Biological Revolution in Psychiatry. New York, Harper and Row, 1984

Burns D: Feeling Good: The New Mood Therapy. New York, William Morrow and Company, 1980

Fieve RR: Moodswing: The Third Revolution in Psychiatry. New York, Bantam, 1976

Kline NS: From Sad to Glad. New York, Ballantine, 1981

Korpell HS: How You Can Help: A Guide for Families of Psychiatric Hospital Patients. Washington, DC, American Psychiatric Press, 1984

Mendelson JH, Mello NK: Alcohol Use and Abuse in America. Boston, Little, Brown, 1985

The Pill Book of Anxiety and Depression. New York, Bantam, 1986

Pope HG, Hudson JI: New Hope for Binge Eaters. New York, Harper and Row, 1984

Schou M: Lithium Treatment of Manic-Depressive Illness, 2nd ed. Basel, S. Karger, 1983

Sheehan DV: The Anxiety Disease and How to Overcome It. New York, Scribner, 1984

Tsuang MT: Schizophrenia: The Facts. New York, Oxford University Press, 1982

Winokur G: Depression: The Facts. New York, Oxford University Press, 1981

Index

I